Contents

Qualitative research in health care

Third edition

Edited by

Catherine Pope
Nicholas Mays

Blackwell
Publishing

Blackwell Publishing, Inc., 350 Main Street, Malden, Massachusetts 02148-5020, USA
Blackwell Publishing Ltd, 9600 Garsington Road, Oxford OX4 2DQ, UK
Blackwell Publishing Asia Pty Ltd, 550 Swanston Street, Carlton, Victoria 3053, Australia

First published 1996 by BMJ Publishing Group
Second edition 1999 by BMJ Publishing Group
Third edition 2006

2   2008

Library of Congress Cataloging-in-Publication Data

Qualitative research in health care/edited by Catherine Pope and
    Nicholas Mays. – 3rd ed.
      p. ; cm.
    Includes bibliographical references and index.
    ISBN: 978-1-4051-3512-2 (alk. paper)
    1. Medical care–Research–Methodology. 2. Qualitative research.
I. Pope, Catherine. II. Mays, Nicholas.
    [DNLM: 1. Health Services Research–methods. 2. Focus Groups.
3. Interviews. 4. Quality Assurance, Health Care. 5. Research
Design. W 84.3 Q18 2006]
RA440.85.Q35 2006
362.1072–dc22

                                                    2006000963

A catalogue record for this title is available from the British Library

Set in 9.25/12 pt Meridien by Newgen Imaging Systems (P) Ltd., Chennai, India

Commissioning Editor: Mary Banks
Editorial Assistant: Vicky Pittman
Development Editor: Vicki Donald
Production Controller: Debbie Wyer

For further information on Blackwell Publishing, visit our website:
www.blackwellpublishing.com

List of contributors

Editors

Catherine Pope, School of Nursing and Midwifery, University of Southampton, Southampton, UK

Nicholas Mays, London School of Hygiene & Tropical Medicine, London, UK

Contributors

Nick Black, London School of Hygiene & Tropical Medicine, London, UK

Nicky Britten, Institute of Health and Social Care Research, Peninsula Medical School, Universities of Exeter and Plymouth, Exeter, UK

Sarah Collins, Department of Health Sciences and Hull/York Medical School, University of York, York, UK

Dawn Goodwin, Institute for Health Research, Lancaster University, Lancaster, UK

Justin Keen, Institute of Health Sciences and Public Health Research, University of Leeds, Leeds, UK

Jenny Kitzinger, Cardiff School of Journalism, Media and Cultural Studies, Cardiff University, Cardiff, UK

Julienne Meyer, Department of Adult Nursing, St. Bartholomew School of Nursing & Midwifery, City University, London, UK

Alicia O'Cathain, School of Health and Related Research, University of Sheffield, Sheffield, UK

Kate Thomas, School of Healthcare, University of Leeds, Leeds, UK

Sue Ziebland, Department of Primary Healthcare, University of Oxford, Oxford, UK

Preface

We had no idea in 1996 that we would, a decade later, be embarking on a third edition of this book. When we wrote the original paper [1] which inspired the book, qualitative methods were largely unfamiliar to health professionals and researchers, but the intervening years have seen a huge expansion in the use of these methods in health care research. The place of qualitative research is now sufficiently recognised at the highest level to merit the commissioning, by the UK Cabinet Office, of a guide for civil servants and researchers on how to assess the quality of qualitative policy evaluations [2].

Having begun life as a series of papers in the *British Medical Journal*, this book has become international – having been translated into Japanese and Portuguese [3,4] – and we find that its readership now includes health care professionals working in different health systems, researchers from diverse disciplinary backgrounds, and policy makers and research funders from across the globe. This book is now one of several on the application of qualitative research to health care, but we believe that it remains distinctive as a way into the field for those with little or no previous knowledge of qualitative methods.

For the third edition we have updated the existing material, incorporating new examples and references, and added new chapters on topics that we see as increasingly relevant in an introductory text. As well as introducing the key methods the book now includes chapters exploring the interface between qualitative and quantitative research – in primary 'mixed method' studies and in the emerging arena of secondary analysis and 'research synthesis'. We owe a debt of thanks to all the authors – those who contributed to the previous editions and those involved in producing this volume – for making the editing process so straightforward for us.

As ever this book has been improved by the constructive advice, commentary and expertise of colleagues, readers and reviewers. Other researchers have made our job easier by opening up and contributing to debates about methodology and research quality, and by simply undertaking the kinds of qualitative research that we refer to in this book. We remain grateful to our editorial team: Mary Banks who has supported us since the first edition, and the new team at Blackwell Publishing, notably Vicki Donald.

Catherine Pope and Nicholas Mays, 2006

References

1. Pope C & Mays N. Opening the black box: an encounter in the corridors of health services research. *British Medical Journal* 1993; **306**: 315–318.
2. Spencer L, Ritchie J, Lewis J *et al. Quality in Qualitative Evaluation: A Framework for Assessing Research Evidence.* Government Chief Social Researcher's Office, Prime Minister's Strategy Unit, Cabinet Office, London, 2003. http://www.strategy.gov.uk
3. Pope C & Mays N. *Qualitative Research in Health Care.* Ikakju-Shoin Ltd, Tokyo, 2001.
4. Pope C & Mays N. *Pesquisa qualitative an atenção à saúde.* (translated by Ananyr Porto Fajardo). Artmed, Porto Alegra, 2005.

CHAPTER 1

Qualitative methods in health research

Catherine Pope, Nicholas Mays

Qualitative methods have much to offer those studying health care and health services. However, because these methods have traditionally been employed in the social sciences, they may be unfamiliar to health care professionals and researchers with a biomedical or natural science background. Indeed, qualitative methods may seem alien alongside the experimental and observational quantitative methods used in clinical, biological and epidemiological research.

Misunderstandings about the nature of qualitative methods and their uses have caused qualitative research to be labelled 'unscientific', difficult to replicate or as little more than anecdote, personal impression or conjecture. The first edition of this book, and the series of papers in the *British Medical Journal* on which the book was initially based, deliberately set out to counter this view. The growing interest in qualitative methods in health research, and their increasing acceptance in clinical and biomedical arenas, in the 10 years since the book was first published, suggest that such misunderstandings may be diminishing. The purpose of this book has therefore altered subtly. Its main aim continues to be to introduce the main qualitative methods available for the study of health and health care, and to show how qualitative research can be employed appropriately and fruitfully to answer some of the increasingly complex questions confronting researchers. In addition, the book considers the ethics of qualitative research and how to assess its quality and looks at the application of qualitative methods within different styles of research and in the emerging area of research synthesis.

The link between theory and method

Some of the earlier misunderstandings about qualitative research were compounded by some of the terminology used, which was, and may still be, unfamiliar to researchers who do not have a social science background. The terms 'qualitative research' and 'qualitative methods' are often used interchangeably, but, strictly speaking, the term *research methods* refer to specific research techniques used to gather data about the social world. The choice of research method is typically informed by a *research strategy* or a set of decisions about the research design, and by beliefs about how the social world can be studied and how the validity of social knowledge established by such research might be assessed. For many social scientists, the choice of a particular research method is also inextricably linked to a particular *theoretical perspective*, or set of explanatory concepts, that provide a framework for thinking about the social world and inform their research (see Box 1.1).

As a result of these different theoretical positions, qualitative research is neither unified nor well defined. There is considerable debate about what constitutes the central tenet of qualitative research. So, for example, Silverman [3] reviews four 'definitions' of qualitative research before offering his own prescriptive account of what qualitative research should be. Elsewhere, Hammersley [4] has examined the methodological ideas that underlie the distinctive Chicagoan tradition of qualitative research, with its emphasis on naturalistic methods (see below). The debate about qualitative research is such that Denzin and Lincoln [5] are forced to conclude that it is 'defined primarily by a series of essential tensions, contradictions and hesitations'. The distinctions between the various theoretical stances are frequently presented as clear-cut, but in practice the contrasts are often less apparent. Moreover, the connection

---

Box 1.1 Some theoretical perspectives that inform qualitative methods [1,2]

- Ethnography
- Symbolic interactionism
- Constructionism
- Ethnomethodology
- Phenomenology

between research and theoretical perspective may not always be clear: sometimes the link is implicit or is simply not acknowledged. So, while many social scientists contend that research should be theoretically driven, others have suggested that the link between theory and methods is overstated. Brannen, for example, has argued that

> the practice of research is a messy untidy business which rarely conforms to the models set down in methodology textbooks. In practice it is unusual, for example, for epistemology (i.e. the specific theory of the nature of knowledge adopted by the researcher) to be the sole determinant of method... There is no necessary or one-to-one correspondence between epistemology and methods [6: 3,15].

She suggests that the choice of method and how it is used are as likely to be informed by the research question or pragmatic or technical considerations as by the researcher's theoretical stance (though others would disagree). This may be particularly the case in health services research because of its applied nature: research here tends to be geared towards specific practical problems or issues and this, rather than theoretical leanings, may determine the methods employed.

So what is qualitative research?

Qualitative research is often defined by reference to quantitative research. Indeed, the articles on which the first edition of this book was based were commissioned, not as a series about qualitative research, but as a series on 'non-quantitative methods'. An unfortunate corollary of this way of defining qualitative research is the inference that because qualitative research does not seek to quantify or enumerate, it does not 'measure'. It is worth noting that it is both feasible and legitimate to analyse certain types of qualitative data quantitatively (see Chapter 7). Whilst it is true that qualitative research generally deals with talk or words rather than numbers, this does not mean that it is devoid of measurement, or that it cannot be used to explain social phenomena.

Measurement in qualitative research is usually concerned with *taxonomy* or classification. Qualitative research answers questions such as, 'what is X, and how does X vary in different circumstances, and why?' rather than 'how big is X or how many X's are there?'

It is concerned with the meanings people attach to their experiences of the social world and how they make sense of that world. It therefore tries to interpret social phenomena (interactions, behaviours, etc.) in terms of the meanings people bring to them; because of this it is often referred to as *interpretative* research. This approach means that the researcher frequently has to question common sense assumptions or ideas that are taken for granted. Bauman, talking about sociology in general, refers to this as 'defamiliarising' [7] and this is just what qualitative research tries to do. Rather than simply accepting the concepts and explanations used in everyday life, qualitative research asks fundamental and searching questions about the nature of social phenomena. So, for example, instead of counting the number of suicides, which presumes that we already agree on the nature of suicide, the researcher may well start by asking, 'what is suicide and how is it defined in this society?' and go on to show that it is socially constructed by the activities of coroners, legal experts, health professionals and individuals, so that definitions of suicide vary considerably between different countries, different cultures and religious groups, and across time [8].

A second distinguishing feature of qualitative research, and one of its key strengths, is that it studies people in their natural settings rather than in artificial or experimental ones. Kirk and Miller define qualitative research as a 'particular tradition in social science that fundamentally depends on watching people in their own territory, and interacting with them in their own language, on their own terms' [9: 9]. This is referred to as *naturalism* – hence the term *naturalistic methods* that is sometimes used to denote the approach used in much, but not all, qualitative research.

Another feature of qualitative research (which some authors emphasise) is that it often employs several different qualitative methods. Watching people in their own territory can thus entail observing, joining in (*participant observation*), talking to people (interviews, focus groups and informal chatting) and reading what they have written. In the health care context, a range of qualitative research methods has been employed to tackle important questions about social phenomena, ranging from complex human behaviours such as patients' compliance with treatment [10], and decision making by health care professionals [11], through to the organisation of the hospital clinic [12] or of the health system as a whole [13,14].

Qualitative research, thus defined, appears very different from quantitative research. Much is made of the differences between the two. The so-called qualitative–quantitative divide is often reinforced by highlighting a corresponding split in the social sciences between social theories concerned with delineating social structure and those concerned with understanding social action or meaning [15,16]. The crude alignment of qualitative research with 'action' or interpretive approaches and quantitative research with 'structural' or positivist ones has meant that researchers on either side have tended to become locked into adversarial positions, ignorant of each other's work. The differences between qualitative and quantitative research are, as a result, frequently overstated, and this has helped to perpetuate the misunderstanding of qualitative methods within such fields as health services research [17]. However, there is a growing recognition within sociology that the qualitative–quantitative distinction may not be helpful or even accurate [18,19]. In the context of health and health services research qualitative and quantitative methods are increasingly being used together in mixed method approaches (see Chapter 9 for more on this) [20].

The uses of qualitative research

Quantitative and qualitative approaches can complement each other. One simple way in which this can be achieved is by using qualitative research as the preliminary to quantitative research. This model is likely to be the most familiar to those engaged in health and health services research. For example, qualitative research can classify phenomena, or answer the 'what is X?' question, which necessarily precedes the process of enumeration of X's. As health care deals with people and people are, on the whole, more complex than the subjects of the natural sciences, there is a whole set of such questions about human interaction, and how people interpret interaction, to which health professionals may need answers before attempting to quantify behaviours or events. At their most basic, qualitative research techniques can be used simply to discover the most comprehensible terms or words in common use to include in a subsequent survey questionnaire. An excellent example of this can be found in the preliminary work undertaken for the British national survey of sexual attitudes and lifestyles [21]. In this case, face-to-face interviews were used to uncover popular ambiguities and misunderstandings in the use of a number of terms such as 'vaginal sex', 'oral sex', 'penetrative sex' and 'heterosexual'. This qualitative work had enormous value in informing the development of the subsequent survey questionnaire, and in ensuring the validity of the data obtained because the language in the questionnaire was clear and could be widely understood.

Qualitative research is not only useful as the first stage of quantitative research. It also has a role to play in 'validating' quantitative research or in providing a different perspective on the same social phenomena. Sometimes it can force a major reinterpretation of quantitative data. For example, one anthropological study using qualitative methods uncovered the severe limitations of previous surveys: Stone and Campbell found that cultural traditions and unfamiliarity with questionnaires had led Nepalese villagers to feign ignorance of abortion and family planning services, and to under-report their use of contraception and abortion when responding to surveys [22]. More often, the insights provided by qualitative research help to interpret or understand quantitative data more fully. Bloor's work on the surgical decision making process built on an epidemiological study of the widespread variations in rates of common surgical procedures (see Box 1.2) and helped to unpack the reasons why these variations occurred [11]. Elsewhere, Morgan and Watkin's research on cultural beliefs about hypertension has helped to explain why rates of compliance with prescribed medications vary significantly amongst and between white and Afro-Caribbean patients [10].

As well as complementing quantitative work, qualitative research may be used quite independently to uncover social processes, or access areas of social life that are not open or amenable to quantitative research. This type of 'stand alone' qualitative research is increasingly being used in studies of health service organisation and policy. It has been used to considerable effect in evaluating organisational reforms and changes to health service provision from the viewpoint of patients, health professionals and managers [14,23]. This type of research has also been useful in examining how data about health and health care are shaped by the social processes that produce them – from waiting lists [24] to death certificates [25] and AIDS registrations [26].

Methods used in qualitative research

Qualitative research explores people's subjective understandings of their everyday lives. Although the different social science disciplines use qualitative methods in slightly different ways, broadly speaking,

Box 1.2 Two-stage investigation of the association between differences in geographic incidence of operations on the tonsils and adenoids and local differences in specialists' clinical practices [27]

I **Epidemiological study – documenting variations**
Analysis of 12 months' routine data on referral, acceptance, and operation rates for new patients under 15 years in two Scottish regions known to have significantly different 10-year operation rates for tonsils and adenoids.

Found significant differences between similar areas within regions in referral, acceptance, and operation rates that were not explained by disease incidence.

Operation rates influenced, in order of importance, by:
• Differences between specialists in propensity to list for operations
• Differences between GPs in propensity to refer
• Differences between areas in symptomatic mix of referrals.

II **Sociological study – explaining how and why variations come about.** Observation of assessment routines undertaken in outpatient departments by six consultants in each region on a total of 493 patients under 15 years
Found considerable variation between specialists in their assessment practices (search procedures and decision rules), which led to differences in disposals, which in turn created local variations in surgical incidence.

'High operators' tended to view a broad spectrum of clinical signs as important and tended to assert the importance of examination findings over the child's history; 'low operators' gave the examination less weight in deciding on disposal and tended to judge a narrower range of clinical features as indicating the need to operate.

the methods used in qualitative research include direct observation, interviews, the analysis of texts or documents and the analysis of recorded speech or behaviour using audio or video tapes. Data collected by these methods may be used differently (e.g. semiotics and psychotherapy both use video and audio-taped material, but their analytical approaches are distinctive), but there is a common focus on talk and action rather than numbers. On one level, these 'qualitative methods' are used every day by human beings to make sense of the world – we watch what is going on, ask questions of each other and try to comprehend the social world we live in. The key difference between these and the qualitative methods employed in social science is that the latter are explicit and systematic. Qualitative research, therefore, involves the application of logical, planned and thorough methods of collecting data, and careful, thoughtful and, above all, rigorous analysis. As several recent commentators have pointed out, this means that qualitative research requires considerable skill on the part of the researcher [28,29]. Perhaps more than some quantitative research techniques, qualitative research needs experienced researchers. One of the problems arising from the rapid expansion of qualitative methods into medical and health fields is that the necessary skill and experience are sometimes lacking.

This book focuses on ways of doing qualitative research which, in essence, rely on conversation (talking) and/or observation (watching). Qualitative researchers use conversation, in the form of interviews, to collect data about people's views and experiences. Interviews can be individual or focus groups (group interviews) (Chapters 2 and 3). In addition, talk or conversation can be analysed in much greater detail using an approach called conversation analysis (Chapter 5). Observation (Chapter 4) is used to collect information about behaviour and events, but may also involve collecting examples of how people talk (e.g. their attitudes to, and understandings of, issues). The book concentrates on these methods because they appear to be the most widely used in health and health services settings. We have neglected documentary methods and forms of textual analysis [30], which have been used in the health field, for example, to describe mass media reporting of AIDS [31], to ascertain the public and professional attitudes to tranquilliser use portrayed by the popular press [32], and to study diaries kept by rural dwellers during the UK foot and mouth disease outbreak of 2001 [33].

The book is introductory and aims to show how these methods can be employed in health research. It seeks to provide clear examples of these methods and to indicate some of the benefits and common pitfalls in their use. It is not a substitute for seeking the advice of a skilled, experienced researcher, nor is it an exhaustive manual for qualitative research. In addition to the references, which provide a route to more detailed material on each of the topics covered, each chapter ends with a short guide to further reading that would be well worth doing before planning a study or going into the field. Chapter 6 provides an introduction to some of the key ethical issues confronting qualitative research, and again this is not intended as exhaustive, but rather to illustrate some of the special dilemmas encountered when doing qualitative research. Chapter 7 outlines how qualitative data are analysed and includes a description of the main software packages currently available to assist this process. Chapter 8 examines the issue of 'quality' in qualitative research and how it may be assessed and assured. Chapters 9–12 explore some of the ways in which qualitative methods are applied in health research. We have chosen examples (mixed methods, case studies, action research, and consensus development,) where qualitative methods are currently used in health and health services research simply to demonstrate how qualitative methods may be used. It is not our intention to argue that these approaches are synonymous with the whole of qualitative research, but rather to indicate that qualitative methods have fruitfully been employed in these ways. The final chapter introduces research synthesis and looks at the ways in which qualitative methods are being employed to integrate research evidence in health and health care.

Further reading

Green J & Thorogood N. *Qualitative Methods for Health Research.* SAGE, London, 2004.

Murphy E, Dingwall R, Greatbatch D, Parker S & Watson P. Qualitative research methods in health technology assessment: a review of the literature. *Health Technology Assessment* 1998; **2**(16) (see section 1).

References

1. Marshall C & Rossman G. *Designing Qualitative Research.* SAGE, London, 1989.
2. Feldman MS. *Strategies for Interpreting Qualitative Data.* Qualitative Research Methods Series, No 33. SAGE, Thousand Oaks, CA, 1995.
3. Silverman D. *Interpreting Qualitative Data: Methods for Analysing Talk, Text and Interaction.* SAGE, London, 1993.
4. Hammersley M. *The Dilemma of Qualitative Method: Herbert Blumer and The Chicago Tradition.* Routledge, London, 1989.
5. Denzin NK & Lincoln YS, eds. *Handbook of Qualitative Research.* SAGE, London, 1994: ix.

6. Brannen J, ed. *Mixing Methods: Qualitative and Quantitative Research.* Avebury, Aldershot, 1992: 3, 15.
7. Bauman Z. *Thinking Sociologically.* Blackwell, Oxford, 1990.
8. Douglas J. *The Social Meanings of Suicide.* Princeton University Press, Princeton, NJ, 1967.
9. Kirk J & Miller M. *Reliability and Validity in Qualitative Research.* Qualitative Research Methods Series, No 1. SAGE, London, 1986: 9.
10. Morgan M & Watkins C. Managing hypertension: beliefs and responses to medication among cultural groups. *Sociology of Health and Illness* 1988; **10**: 561–578.
11. Bloor M. Bishop Berkeley and the adenotonsillectomy enigma: an exploration of the social construction of medical disposals. *Sociology* 1976; **10**: 43–61.
12. Strong PM. *The Ceremonial Order of the Clinic.* Routledge, London, 1979.
13. Strong PM & Robinson J. *The NHS: Under New Management.* Open University Press, Milton Keynes, 1990.
14. Pollitt C, Harrison S, Hunter D *et al.* General management in the NHS: the initial impact, 1983–88. *Public Administration* 1991; **69**: 61–83.
15. Mechanic D. Medical sociology: some tensions among theory, method and substance. *Journal of Health and Social Behavior* 1989; **30**: 147–160.
16. Pearlin L. Structure and meaning in medical sociology. *Journal of Health and Social Behavior* 1992; **33**: 1–9.
17. Pope C & Mays N. Opening the black box: an encounter in the corridors of health services research. *British Medical Journal* 1990; **306**: 315–318.
18. Abell P. Methodological achievements in sociology over the past few decades with special reference to the interplay of qualitative and quantitative methods. In: Bryant C & Becker H, eds. *What Has Sociology Achieved?* Macmillan, London, 1990.
19. Hammersley M. Deconstructing the qualitative-quantitative divide. In: Brannen J, ed. *Mixing Methods: Qualitative and Quantitative Research.* Avebury, Aldershot, 1992.
20. Barbour R. The case for combining qualitative and quantitative approaches in health services research. *Journal of Health Services Research and Policy* 1999; **4**: 39–43.
21. Wellings K, Field J, Johnson A *et al. Sexual Behaviour in Britain: The National Survey of Sexual Attitudes and Lifestyles.* Penguin, Harmondsworth, 1994.
22. Stone L & Campbell JG. The use and misuse of surveys in international development: an experiment from Nepal. *Human Organisation* 1986; **43**: 27–37.
23. Packwood T, Keen J & Buxton M. *Hospitals in Transition: The Resource Management Experiment.* Open University Press, Milton Keynes, 1991.

24. Pope C. Trouble in store: some thoughts on the management of waiting lists. *Sociology of Health and Illness* 1991; **13**: 191–211.
25. Prior L & Bloor M. Why people die: social representations of death and its causes. *Science As Culture* 1993; **3**: 346–374.
26. Bloor M, Goldberg D & Emslie J. Ethnostatistics and the AIDS epidemic. *British Journal of Sociology* 1991; **42**: 131–137.
27. Bloor MJ, Venters GA & Samphier ML. Geographical variation in the incidence of operations on the tonsils and adenoids: an epidemiological and sociological investigation. *Journal of Laryngol and Otology* 1976; **92**: 791–801, 883–895.
28. Malterud K. Shared understanding of the qualitative research process: guidelines for the medical researcher. *Family Practice* 1993; **10**: 201–206.
29. Dingwall R, Murphy E, Watson P *et al.* Catching goldfish: quality in qualitative research. *Journal of Health Services Research and Policy* 1998; **3**: 167–172.
30. Plummer K. *Documents of Life: An Introduction to Problems and Literature of a Humanistic Method.* Allen and Unwin, London, 1983.
31. Kitzinger J & Miller D. "African AIDS": the media an audience believes. In: Aggleton P, Davies P & Hart G, eds. *AIDS: Rights, Risk and Reason.* Falmer Press, London, 1992.
32. Gabe J, Gustaffson U & Bury M. Mediating illness: newspaper coverage of tranquilliser dependence. *Sociology of Health and Illness* 1991; **13**: 332–353.
33. Mort M, Convery I, Baxter J *et al.* Psychosocial effects of the 2001 UK foot and mouth disease epidemic in a rural population: qualitative diary based study. *British Medical Journal* 2005; **331**: 1234–1238.

CHAPTER 2
Qualitative interviews

Nicky Britten

Interviews are the most commonly used qualitative technique in health care settings. The attraction of interview-based studies for practising clinicians is their apparent proximity to the clinical task. However, this is also a danger as the many differences between clinical work and qualitative research may be overlooked.

Types of qualitative interview

Practising clinicians routinely interview patients during their clinical work, and they may wonder whether simply talking to people constitutes a legitimate form of research. In sociology and related disciplines, however, interviewing is a well-established research technique. There are three main types: structured, semistructured and depth interviews (see Box 2.1).

Structured interviews consist of administering structured questionnaires, and interviewers are trained to ask questions (mostly with a fixed choice of responses) in a standardised manner. For example, interviewees might be asked: 'Is your health excellent, good, fair or poor?' Though qualitative interviews are often described as being

---

Box 2.1 Types of interviews

- Structured
    Usually with a structured questionnaire
- Semistructured
    Open ended questions
- Depth
    One or two issues covered in great detail
    Questions are based on what the interviewee says

---

unstructured to contrast them with this type of formalised interview designed to yield quantitative data, the term 'unstructured' is misleading, as no interview is completely devoid of structure. If there were no structure, there would be no guarantee that the data gathered would be appropriate to the research question.

Semistructured interviews are conducted on the basis of a loose structure consisting of open-ended questions that define the area to be explored, at least initially, and from which the interviewer or interviewee may diverge to pursue an idea or response in more detail. Continuing with the same example, interviewees might initially be asked a series of questions such as: 'What do you think good health is?', 'How do you consider your own health?' and so on.

Depth interviews are less structured than this, and may cover only one or two issues, but in much greater detail. Such an interview might begin with the interviewer saying, 'This research study is about how people think about their own health. Can you tell me about your own health experiences?' Further questions from the interviewer would be based on what the interviewee said, and would consist mostly of clarification and probing for details.

Interviews have been used extensively in studies of both patients and doctors. For example, Townsend *et al.* interviewed 23 men and women aged about 50 years with four or more chronic illnesses on two separate occasions [1]. Interviews were semistructured, but interviewees were encouraged to talk freely about their experiences and management strategies for their conditions. The data revealed that interviewees expressed ambivalence to taking drugs in several ways. Drugs both enabled interviewees to continue to function in social roles and acted as a marker of their inability to perform such roles. Huby *et al.* interviewed 26 general practitioners about their experiences of well being and distress at work, and the relation between work and home [2]. They found that morale in general practice depended on several factors; the dynamics of the relations between the factors was more important than any one factor in isolation. Practice partnership arrangements were a key factor in mediating between external workload pressures and individual general practitioners' experience of work.

Clinical and qualitative research interviews have very different purposes. Although the doctor may be willing to see the problem from the patient's perspective, the clinical task is to fit that problem into an appropriate medical category to choose an appropriate form of management. The constraints of most consultations are such that any open-ended questioning needs to be brought to a conclusion by the doctor within a fairly short time. In a qualitative research interview, the aim is to discover the interviewee's own framework of meanings and the research task is to avoid imposing the researcher's structures and assumptions on the interviewee's account as far as possible. The researcher needs to remain open to the possibility that the concepts and variables that emerge may be very different from those that might have been predicted at the outset.

Qualitative interview studies address different questions from those addressed by quantitative research. For example, a quantitative study might measure age-standardised admission rates for asthma for black and south Asian patients compared with white patients. In a qualitative study, by contrast, Griffiths *et al.* interviewed south Asian and white adults with asthma to explore their experiences of hospital admission and contributing factors, coping with asthma, causes of exacerbations, and relationships with clinicians [3]. In a longitudinal qualitative study of people with chronic illness having acupuncture for the first time, Paterson and Britten asked about interviewees' responses to three standardised health status questionnaires [4]. The questionnaires varied in their ability to reflect and measure changes that were important to interviewees. Qualitative research can also open up different areas of research such as patients' use of the internet [5], or the ways in which patients recruited to clinical trials understand concepts such as 'trial' or 'watchful waiting'. In Donovan *et al.*'s study, some patients interpreted 'watchful waiting' to mean that clinicians would 'watch while I die' [6: 768].

Conducting interviews

Qualitative interviewers try to be interactive and sensitive to the language and concepts used by the interviewee, and they try to keep the agenda flexible. They aim to go below the surface of the topic being discussed, explore what people say in as much detail as possible, and uncover new areas or ideas that were not anticipated at the outset of the research. It is vital that interviewers check that they have understood respondents' meanings instead of relying on their own assumptions. This is particularly important if there is obvious potential for misunderstanding – for example, when a clinician interviews someone unfamiliar with medical terminology. Clinicians should not assume that interviewees use medical terminology in the same way that they do.

Patton wrote that good questions in qualitative interviews should be open-ended, neutral, sensitive and clear to the interviewee [7]. He listed six types of questions that can be asked: those based on behaviour or experience, on opinion or value, on feeling, on knowledge, on sensory experience, and those asking about demographic or background details (see Box 2.2). It is usually best to start with questions that the interviewee can answer easily and then proceed to more difficult or sensitive topics. Most interviewees are willing to provide the kind of information the researcher wants, but they need to be given clear guidance about the amount of detail required. This way, it is possible to collect data even in stressful circumstances [8].

The less structured the interview, the less the questions are determined and standardised before the interview occurs. Most qualitative interviewers will have an interview schedule that defines the areas to be covered, based on the objectives of their study. Unlike quantitative interviews based on highly structured questionnaires, the order in which questions are asked will vary, as will the questions designed to probe the interviewee's meanings. Wordings cannot be standardised because the interviewer will try to use the person's own vocabulary when framing supplementary questions. Also, during the course of a qualitative study, the interviewer may introduce further questions as he or she becomes more familiar with the topic being discussed.

All qualitative researchers need to consider how they are perceived by interviewees and the effects of personal characteristics such as class, race, sex and social distance on the interview. This question becomes more acute if the interviewee knows that the interviewer is also a doctor or nurse. An interviewee who is already

---

Box 2.2 Types of questions for qualitative interview

- Behaviour or experience
- Opinion or belief
- Feelings
- Knowledge
- Sensory
- Background or demographic

a patient or likely to become one may wish to please the doctor or nurse by giving the responses he or she thinks the doctor or nurse wants. It is best not to interview one's own patients for research purposes, but if this cannot be avoided, patients should be given permission to say what they really think, and they should not be corrected if they say things that clinicians think are wrong (e.g. that antibiotics are a suitable treatment for viral infections).

Interviewers are also likely to be asked questions by interviewees during the course of an interview. The problem with this is that in answering questions, clinical researchers may undo earlier efforts not to impose their own concepts on the interview. On the other hand, if questions are not answered, this may reduce the interviewee's willingness to answer the interviewer's subsequent questions. One solution is to say that such questions can be answered at the end of the interview, although this is not always a satisfactory response [9].

Researcher as research instrument

Qualitative interviews require considerable skill on the part of the interviewer. Experienced doctors and other clinicians may feel that they already possess the necessary skills, and indeed many are transferable. To achieve the transition from consultation to research interview, clinical researchers need to monitor their own interviewing technique, critically appraising tape recordings of their interviews and asking others for their comments. The novice research interviewer needs to notice how directive he or she is being, whether leading questions are being asked, whether cues are picked up or ignored, and whether interviewees are given enough time to explain what they mean. Whyte devised a six-point directiveness scale to help novice researchers analyse their own interviewing technique (see Box 2.3) [10]. The point is not that non-directiveness is always best, but that the amount of directiveness should be appropriate to the style of research. Some informants are more verbose than others, and it is vital that interviewers maintain control of the interview. Patton provided three strategies for maintaining control: knowing the purpose of the interview, asking the right questions to get the information needed, and giving appropriate verbal and non-verbal feedback (see Box 2.4) [7].

Holstein and Gubrium have written about the 'active' interview to emphasise the point that all interviews are collaborative

Box 2.3 Whyte's directiveness scale for analysing interviewing technique [10]

1. Making encouraging noises
2. Reflecting on remarks made by the informant
3. Probing on the last remark by the informant
4. Probing an idea preceding the last remark by the informant
5. Probing an idea expressed earlier in the interview
6. Introducing a new topic
   (1 = least directive, 6 = most directive)

Box 2.4 Maintaining control of the interview [7]

- Knowing what it is you want to find out
- Asking the right questions to get the information you need
- Giving appropriate verbal and non-verbal feedback

enterprises [11]. They argue that both interviewer and interviewee are engaged in the business of constructing meaning, whether this is acknowledged or not. They criticise the traditional view in which a passive respondent accesses a 'vessel of answers' that exists independently of the interview process. The interview is an active process in which the respondent activates different aspects of her or his stock of knowledge with the interviewer's help. They conclude that an active interview study has two aims: 'to gather information about *what* the research project is about and to explicate *how* knowledge concerning that topic is narratively constructed'.

Some common pitfalls for interviewers identified by Field and Morse include outside interruptions, competing distractions, stage fright, awkward questions, jumping from one subject to another, and the temptation to counsel interviewees (see Box 2.5) [12]. Awareness of these pitfalls can help the interviewer to develop ways of overcoming them, ranging from simple tasks such as unplugging the telephone and rephrasing potentially embarrassing questions, through to conducting the interview at the interviewee's own pace and assuring the interviewee that there is no hurry.

Box 2.5 Common pitfalls in interviewing [12]

- Interruptions from outside (e.g. telephones)
- Competing distractions (e.g. televisions)
- Stage fright for interviewer or interviewee
- Asking interviewee embarrassing or awkward questions
- Jumping from one subject to another
- Teaching (e.g. giving interviewee medical advice)
- Counselling (e.g. summarising responses too early)
- Presenting one's own perspective, thus potentially biasing the interview
- Superficial interviews
- Receiving secret information (e.g. suicide threats)
- Translators (e.g. inaccuracy)

Recording interviews

There are various ways of recording qualitative interviews: notes written at the time, notes written afterwards and audio recording. Writing notes at the time can interfere with the process of interviewing, and notes written afterwards are likely to miss out some details. In certain situations, written notes are preferable to audio recording, but most people will agree to having an interview recorded, although it may take them a little while to speak freely in front of a machine. It is vitally important to use good quality equipment that has been tested beforehand and with which the interviewer is familiar. Digital equipment provides digital files that can then be emailed to co-researchers or to transcribers. Transcription is an immensely time consuming process, as each hour's worth of a one-to-one interview can take six or seven hours to transcribe, depending on the quality of the recording (and, as Chapter 3 explains, this transcription time increases considerably for group interviews). The costing of any interview-based study should include adequate transcription time.

Identifying interviewees

Sampling strategies should always be determined by the purpose of the research project. Statistical representativeness is not normally sought in qualitative research (see Chapter 8 for more on sampling).

Similarly, sample sizes are not determined by hard and fast rules, but by other factors, such as the depth and duration required for each interview and how much it is feasible for a single interviewer to undertake. Large qualitative studies do not often interview more than 50 or 60 people, although there are exceptions [13]. Sociologists conducting research in medical settings often have to negotiate access with great care, although this is unlikely to be a problem for clinicians conducting research in their own place of work. Nevertheless, the researcher still needs to approach the potential interviewee and explain the purpose of the research, if appropriate emphasising that a refusal will not affect future treatment. An introductory letter should also explain what is involved and the likely duration of the interview and should give assurances about confidentiality. Interviews should always be conducted at interviewees' convenience, which for people who work during the day will often be in the evening. The setting of an interview affects the content, and it is usually preferable to interview people in their own homes.

Conclusion

Qualitative interviewing is a flexible and powerful tool that can open up many new areas for research. It is worth remembering that answers to interview questions about behaviour will not necessarily correspond with observational studies: what people say they do is not always the same as what they can be observed doing. That said, qualitative interviews can be used to enable practising clinicians to investigate research questions of immediate relevance to their everyday work, which would otherwise be difficult to investigate. Few researchers would consider embarking on a new research technique without some form of training, and training in research interviewing skills is available from universities and specialist research organisations.

Further reading

Green J & Thorogood N. *Qualitative Methods for Health Research.* SAGE, London, 2004.

Kvale S. *InterViews: An Introduction to Qualitative Research Interviewing.* SAGE, London, 1996.

References

1. Townsend A, Hunt K & Wyke S. Managing multiple morbidity in mid-life: a qualitative study of attitudes to drug use. *British Medical Journal* 2003; **327**: 837–841.
2. Huby G, Gerry M, McKinstry B *et al.* Morale among general practitioners: qualitative study exploring relations between partnership arrangements, personal style, and workload. *British Medical Journal* 2002; **325**: 140–144.
3. Griffiths C, Kaur G, Gantley M *et al.* Influences on hospital admission for asthma in south Asian and white adults: qualitative interview study. *British Medical Journal* 2001; **323**: 962–969.
4. Paterson C & Britten N. Acupuncture for people with chronic illness: combining qualitative and quantitative outcome assessment. *The Journal of Alternative and Complementary Medicine* 2003; **9**: 671–681.
5. Ziebland S, Chapple A, Dumelow C *et al.* How the internet affects patients' experience of cancer: a qualitative study. *British Medical Journal* 2004; **328**: 564–569.
6. Donovan J, Mills N, Smith M *et al.* for the Protect Study Group. Improving design and conduct of randomised trials by embedding them in qualitative research: ProtecT (prostrate testing for cancer and treatment) study. *British Medical Journal* 2002; **325**: 766–770.
7. Patton MQ. *How to Use Qualitative Methods in Evaluation.* SAGE, London, 1987: 108–143.
8. Cannon S. Social research in stressful settings: difficulties for the sociologist studying the treatment of breast cancer. *Sociology of Health and Illness* 1989; **11**: 62–77.
9. Oakley A. Interviewing women: a contradiction in terms. In: Roberts H, ed. *Doing Feminist Research.* Routledge and Kegan Paul, London, 1981: 30–61.
10. Whyte WE. Interviewing in field research. In: Burgess RG, ed. *Field Research: A Sourcebook and Field Manual.* George Allen and Unwin, London, 1982: 111–122.
11. Holstein JA & Gubrium JF. *The Active Interview.* SAGE, London, 1995: 56.
12. Field PA & Morse JM. *Nursing Research: The Application of Qualitative Approaches.* Chapman & Hall, London, 1989.
13. Holland J, Ramazanoglu C, Scott S *et al.* Sex, gender and power: young women's sexuality in the shadow of AIDS. *Sociology of Health and Illness* 1990; **12**: 36–50.

CHAPTER 3
Focus groups

Jenny Kitzinger

What are focus groups?

Focus groups are a form of group interview that capitalises on communication between research participants to generate data. Although group interviews are often employed simply as a quick and convenient way to collect data from several people simultaneously, true focus groups are explicitly designed to capitalise on group interaction to provide distinctive types of data. This means that instead of the researcher asking each person to respond to a question in turn, people are encouraged to talk to one another, ask questions, exchange anecdotes and comment on each others' experiences and points of view (see Box 3.1) [1].

Focus groups were originally employed in communication studies to explore the effects of films and television programmes [2]. Not surprisingly, given their history, focus groups are a popular method for assessing health education messages and examining public understandings of illness and of health behaviours [3–7]. They are also used to gain insights into people's experiences of disease and of health services [8,9], as well as exploring the attitudes and needs of staff [10,11]. Focus groups have been used to examine a wide range of issues including, for example, people's attitudes toward smoking [12], understandings of child sexual abuse and associated policy responses [13], the health needs of lesbians [14], ethnic minority views on screening procedures [15], the impact of AIDS health education [16] and women's experiences of breast cancer [17]. Focus groups have also been used to explore issues such as professional responses to changing management arrangements [18] and to find ways of improving medical education and professional development [19].

The idea behind the focus group method is that group processes can help people to explore and clarify their views in ways that would

---

Box 3.1 Interaction between participants can be used:

- to highlight the respondents' attitudes, priorities, language and framework of understanding
- to encourage research participants to generate and explore their own questions, and to develop their own analysis of common experiences
- to encourage a variety of communication from participants – tapping into a wide range and different forms of discourse
- to help to identify group norms/cultural values
- to provide insight into the operation of group social processes in the articulation of knowledge (e.g. through the examination of what information is sensitive within the group)
- to encourage open conversation about embarrassing subjects and to permit the expression of criticism
- generally to facilitate the expression of ideas and experiences that might be left underdeveloped in an interview, and to illuminate the research participants' perspectives through the debate within the group.

---

be less easily accessible in a one-to-one interview. Group discussion is particularly appropriate when the interviewer has a series of open-ended questions and wishes to encourage research participants to explore the issues of importance to them, in their own vocabulary, generating their own questions and pursuing their own priorities. When group dynamics works well the co-participants act as co-researchers, taking the research in new and often unexpected directions.

Group work also helps researchers tap into the many different forms of communication that people use in day-to-day interaction, including jokes, anecdotes, teasing and arguing. Gaining access to such a variety of communication is useful because people's knowledge and attitudes are not entirely encapsulated in reasoned responses to direct questions. Everyday forms of communication may show as much, if not more, about what people know or experience. In this sense, focus groups 'reach the parts that other methods cannot reach', revealing dimensions of understanding that often remain untapped by other forms of data collection.

Tapping into such interpersonal communication is also important because it can highlight (sub)cultural values or group norms.

Through analysing the operation of humour, consensus and dissent, and examining different types of narrative employed within the group, the researcher can identify shared knowledge [20]. This makes the focus group a particularly culturally sensitive data collection technique, which is why it is so often employed in cross-cultural research and work with ethnic minorities. It also makes focus groups useful in studies that examine why different sections of the population make differential use of health services [21]. For similar reasons, focus groups are useful for studying dominant cultural values (e.g. exposing dominant narratives about sexuality) [22] and for examining work place cultures – for example, the ways in which staff cope with the stress of working with terminally ill patients or deal with the pressures of an Accident and Emergency Department.

The presence of other research participants can compromise the usual confidentiality of a research setting, so special care should be taken, especially when working with 'captive' populations (such as patients in a hospice). However, it should not be assumed that groups are always more inhibiting than one-to-one interviews or that focus groups are inappropriate when researching sensitive topics. In fact, quite the opposite may be true. Group work can actively facilitate the discussion of difficult topics because the less inhibited members of the group break the ice for shyer participants [13,14]. Co-participants can also provide mutual support in expressing feelings that are common to their group, but which they consider to deviate from mainstream culture (or the assumed culture of the researcher). This is particularly important when researching taboo or stigmatised experiences (e.g. bereavement or sexual violence).

Focus group methods are also popular with those conducting *action research* (see Chapter 11) and those concerned to empower research participants, who can become an active part of the research development and analysis process [23]. Group participants may develop particular perspectives as a consequence of talking with other people who have similar experiences. For example, group dynamics can allow for a shift from self-blaming psychological explanations ('I'm stupid not to have understood what the doctor was telling me' or 'I should have been stronger – I should have asked the right questions,') to the exploration of structural solutions ('If we've all felt confused about what we've been told maybe having a leaflet would help' or 'What about being able to take away a tape-recording of the consultation?').

Some researchers have also noted that group discussions can generate more critical comments than interviews [24]. Geis and his colleagues, in their study of the lovers of people with AIDS, found that there were more angry comments about the medical community in the group discussions than in the individual interviews: '... perhaps the synergism of the group "kept the anger going" and allowed each participant to reinforce another's vented feelings of frustration and rage...' [25: 43]. Using a method that facilitates the expression of criticism and, at the same time, the exploration of different types of solutions, is invaluable if one is seeking to improve services. Such a method is especially appropriate when working with particularly disempowered patient populations who are often reluctant to give negative feedback [26].

Conducting a focus group study

Sampling and group composition
Focus group studies can consist of anything from half a dozen to over 50 groups, depending on the aims of the project and the resources available. Even just a few discussion sessions can generate a large amount of data, and for this reason many studies rely on a modest number of groups. Some studies combine this method with other data collection techniques; for example, group discussion of a questionnaire is an ideal way of testing out the phrasing of questions for a survey and is also useful when seeking to explain or explore survey results [27,28].

Although it may be possible to work with a representative sample of a small population, most focus group studies use purposive sampling whereby participants are selected to reflect the range within the total study population or theoretical sampling designed to test particular hypotheses. An imaginative approach to sampling is crucial. Most people now recognise social class or ethnicity as important sampling variables. However, it is also worth considering other variables. For example, when exploring women's experiences of maternity care it may be advisable explicitly to include groups of women who were sexually abused as children as they can provide unique insights about respectful care or the power relationships underlying the delivery of care [29].

Most researchers recommend aiming for homogeneity within each group to capitalise on people's shared experiences. However, it can also be advantageous on occasions to bring together a diverse group (e.g. from a range of professions) to maximise exploration of different perspectives within a group setting. However, it is important to be aware of how hierarchy within the group may affect the data. A nursing auxiliary is likely to be inhibited by the presence of a medical specialist from the same hospital, for example.

The groups can be 'naturally occurring', such as people who work together, or may be drawn together specifically for the research. By using pre-existing groups, one is able to observe fragments of interactions that approximate to naturally occurring data (such as might have been collected by participant observation (see Chapter 4 for more on this)). An additional advantage is that friends and colleagues can relate each other's comments to actual incidents in their shared daily lives. They may challenge each other on contradictions between what they profess to believe and how they actually behave (e.g. 'how about that time you didn't use a glove while taking blood from a patient?').

It would be naïve, however, to assume that group data are by definition 'natural' in the sense that such interactions would have occurred without the group being convened for this purpose. Rather than assuming that sessions inevitably reflect everyday interactions (although sometimes they will), the group should be used to encourage people to engage with one another, formulate their ideas and draw out the ways they think about issues that might not have been articulated previously.

Finally, it is important to consider the appropriateness of group work for different study populations and to think about how to overcome potential difficulties. Group work can facilitate collecting information from people who cannot read or write. The 'safety in numbers' factor may also encourage the participation of those who are wary of an interviewer or those who are anxious about talking [30]. However, group work can compound difficulties in communication if each person has a different disability. For example, in a study assessing residential care for the elderly, a focus group was conducted that included one person who had impaired hearing, another with senile dementia and a third with partial paralysis affecting her speech. This severely restricted interaction between research participants and confirmed some of the staff's predictions about the limitations of group work with this population [31]. However, such problems could have been resolved by thinking more carefully about the composition of the group. Sometimes group participants could help to translate for each other, for example. It should also be noted

> **Box 3.2** Some potential sampling advantages of focus groups
>
> - Do not discriminate against people who cannot read or write
> - Can encourage participation from those who are reluctant to be interviewed on their own (such as those intimidated by the formality and isolation of a one-to-one interview)
> - Can encourage contributions from people who feel they have nothing to say or who are deemed 'unresponsive' (but who can engage in the discussion generated by other group members).

that some of the old people who might have been unable to sustain a one-to-one interview were able to take part in the group, contributing intermittently. Even some residents whom staff had suggested should be excluded from the research because they were 'unresponsive' eventually responded to the lively conversations generated by their co-residents and were able to contribute their point of view (see Box 3.2). Considerations of people's diverse communication needs should not rule out group work, but must be considered as a factor.

Running the groups

Sessions should be relaxed: a comfortable setting, refreshments and sitting round in a circle will help to establish the right atmosphere. The ideal group size is from four to eight people. Sessions may last around one or two hours (or extend into a whole afternoon or a series of meetings). The group facilitator should explain that the aim of focus groups is to encourage people to talk to each other rather than to address themselves to the researcher. She/he may take a back seat at first, allowing for a type of 'structured eavesdropping' [32]. Later on in the session, however, the facilitator can adopt a more interventionist style, urging debate to continue beyond the stage at which it might otherwise have ended and encouraging members of the group to discuss the inconsistencies both between participants and within their own thinking.

The facilitator may sometimes take on a 'devil's advocate' role to provoke debate [33]. Disagreements within groups can be used to encourage participants to elucidate their point of view and to clarify why they think as they do. Whereas differences between individual interviewees have to be analysed by the researchers through arm-chair theorising after the event, an advantage of focus groups is that differences between group members can be explored in situ with the help of the research participants.

The facilitator may also take materials along to the group to help to focus and provoke debate [34] such as pictures from the mass media, or advertisements (with their strap lines removed) [35]. Other people take in objects. For example, Chui and Knight passed around a speculum during their group discussions about cervical smears [15], and in Wilkinson's study of breast cancer one woman spontaneously passed around her prosthesis. Such opportunities to see and handle objects not usually available provoked considerable discussion and provided important insights [17].

An alternative or additional type of prompt involves presenting the group with a series of statements on large cards. The group members are asked collectively to sort these cards into different piles depending on, for example, their degree of agreement or disagreement with that point of view or the importance they assign to that particular aspect of service. For example, such cards can be used to explore public understandings of HIV transmission (placing statements about 'types' of people into different risk categories), old people's experiences of residential care (assigning degrees of importance to different statements about the quality of their care), and midwives' views of their professional responsibilities (placing a series of statements about midwives' roles along an agree–disagree continuum). Exercises such as these encourage participants to concentrate on one another (rather than on the group facilitator) and force them to explain their different perspectives. The final layout of the cards is less important than the discussion that it generates. Facilitators may also use this kind of exercise as a way of checking out their own assessment of what has emerged from the group. In this case, it is best to take along a series of blank cards and only fill them out toward the end of the session, using statements generated during the course of the discussion. Finally, it may be beneficial to present research participants with a brief questionnaire, or the opportunity to speak to the facilitator privately, after the group session has been completed.

Ideally the group's discussions should be tape recorded and transcribed. If this is not possible, then it is vital to take careful notes, and researchers may find it useful to involve the group in recording key issues on a flip chart.

Analysis and writing up

The process of analysing qualitative data is discussed in more detail in Chapter 7. Here it is sufficient to note that in analysing focus groups it is particularly important to take full advantage of the data generated through the interaction between research participants. For discussion of different ways of working with focus group data, including using computer-assisted packages, applying conversational or discourse analysis to focus group recordings and transcripts (see Chapter 5 for more on this), or examining 'sensitive moments' in group interaction (see Frankland and Bloor [12], Myers and Macnaghten [36] and Kitzinger and Farquhar [37]).

Conclusion

This chapter has introduced some of the factors to be considered when designing or evaluating a focus group study. In particular, it has drawn attention to the overt exploitation and exploration of interactions in focus group discussion. Group data are neither more nor less authentic than data collected by other methods; rather focus groups may be the most appropriate method for researching particular types of question. Direct observation may be more appropriate for studies of social roles and formal organisations, but focus groups are particularly suited to the study of attitudes and experiences. Interviews may be more appropriate for tapping into individual biographies, but focus groups are more suitable for examining how knowledge and, more importantly, ideas develop, operate and are expressed within a given cultural context. Questionnaires are more appropriate for obtaining quantitative information and explaining how many people hold a certain (pre-defined) opinion. However, focus groups are better for exploring exactly how those opinions are constructed or, depending on your theoretical background, how different 'discourses' are expressed and mobilised (indeed, discourse analysis of focus group data can challenge the idea that 'opinions' exist at all as pre-defined entities to be 'discovered' within individuals) [38].

Focus groups are not an easy option. The data they generate can be complex. Yet, the method is basically straightforward and need not be intimidating for either the researcher or the participants. Perhaps the very best way of working out whether focus groups might be appropriate in any particular study is to read a selection of other people's focus group reports and then to try out a few pilot groups with friends or acquaintances.

Further reading

Barbour R & Kitzinger J. *Developing Focus Group Research: Politics, Theory and Practice.* SAGE, London, 1999.

References

1. Kitzinger J. The methodology of focus groups: the importance of interactions between research participants. *Sociology of Health and Illness* 1994; **16**: 103–121.
2. Merton RK. *The Focused Interview.* Free Press, Glencoe, IL, 1956.
3. Basch C. Focus group interview: an under-utilised research technique for improving theory and practice in health education. *Health Education Quarterly* 1987; **14**: 411–448.
4. Ritchie JE, Herscovitch F & Norfor JB. Beliefs of blue collar workers regarding coronary risk behaviours. *Health Education Research* 1994; **9**: 95–103.
5. Duke SS, Gordon-Sosby K, Reynolds KD *et al.* A study of breast cancer detection practices and beliefs in black women attending public health clinics. *Health Education Research* 1994; **9**: 331–342.
6. Khan M & Manderson L. Focus groups in tropical diseases research. *Health Policy and Planning* 1992; **7**: 56–66.
7. Morgan D. *Focus Groups as Qualitative Research.* SAGE, London, 1988.
8. Murray S, Tapson J, Turnbull L *et al.* Listening to local voices: adapting rapid appraisal to assess health and social needs in general practice. *British Medical Journal* 1994; **308**: 698–700.
9. Gregory S & McKie L. The smear test: listening to women's views. *Nursing Standard* 1991; **5**: 32–36.
10. Brown J, Lent B & Sas G. Identifying and treating wife abuse. *Journal of Family Practice* 1993; **36**: 185–191.
11. Denning JD & Verschelden C. Using the focus group in assessing training needs: empowering child welfare workers. *Child Welfare League of America* 1993; **72**(6): 569–579.
12. Frankland C & Bloor M. Some issues arising in the systematic analysis of focus group materials. In: Barbour R & Kitzinger J, eds. *Developing Focus Group Research: Politics, Theory and Practice.* SAGE, London, 1999.
13. Kitzinger J. *Framing Abuse: Media Influence and Public Understanding of Sexual Violence Against Children.* Pluto, London, 2004.
14. Farquhar C. Are focus groups suitable for 'sensitive' topics? In: Barbour R & Kitzinger J, eds. *Developing Focus Group Research: Politics, Theory and Practice.* SAGE, London, 1999.

15. Chui L & Knight, D. How useful are focus groups for obtaining the views of minority groups? In: Barbour R & Kitzinger J, eds. *Developing Focus Group Research: Politics, Theory and Practice.* SAGE, London, 1999.

16. Kitzinger J. Understanding AIDS: researching audience perceptions of acquired immune deficiency syndrome. In: Eldridge J, ed. *Getting the Message; News, Truth and Power.* Routledge, London, 1993: 271–305.

17. Wilkinson S. Focus groups in health research. *Journal of Health Psychology* 1998; **3**: 323–342.

18. Barbour R. Are focus groups an appropriate tool for studying organisational change? In: Barbour R & Kitzinger J, eds. *Developing Focus Group Research: Politics, Theory and Practice.* SAGE, London, 1999.

19. Barbour, R. Making sense of focus groups. *Medical Education* 2005; **39**(7): 742–750.

20. Hughes D & Dumont K. Using focus groups to facilitate culturally anchored research. *American Journal of Community Psychology* 1993; **21**: 775–806.

21. Naish J, Brown J & Denton, B. Intercultural consultations: investigation of factors that deter non-English speaking women from attending their general practitioners for cervical screening. *British Medical Journal* 1994; **309**: 1126–1128.

22. Barker G & Rich S. Influences on adolescent sexuality in Nigeria and Kenya: findings from recent focus-group discussions. *Studies in Family Planning* 1992; **23**: 199–210.

23. Baker R & Hinton R. Do focus groups facilitate meaningful participation in social research? In: Barbour R & Kitzinger J, eds. *Developing Focus Group Research: Politics, Theory and Practice.* SAGE, London, 1999.

24. Watts M & Ebbutt D. More than the sum of the parts: research methods in group interviewing. *British Educational Research Journal* 1987; **13**: 25–34.

25. Geis S, Fuller R & Rush J. Lovers of AIDS victims: psychosocial stresses and counselling needs. *Death Studies* 1986; **10**: 43–53.

26. DiMatteo M, Kahn K & Berry S. Narratives of birth and the postpartum: an analysis of the focus group responses of new mothers. *Birth* 1993; **20**: 204.

27. Kitzinger J. Focus groups: method or madness? In: Boulton M, ed. *Challenge and Innovation: Methodological Advances in Social Research on HIV/AIDS.* Taylor & Francis, London, 1994: 159–175.

28. O'Brien K. Improving survey questionnaires through focus groups. In: Morgan D, ed. *Successful Focus Groups: Advancing the State of the Art.* SAGE, London, 1993: 105–118.

29. Kitzinger J. Recalling the pain: incest survivors' experiences of obstetrics and gynaecology. *Nursing Times* 1990; **86**: 38–40.

30. Lederman L. High apprehensives talk about communication apprehension and its effects on their behaviour. *Communication Quarterly* 1983; **31**: 233–237.

31. Kitzinger J. Patient Satisfaction survey in the Care of the Elderly Unit, Volume 1: Qualitative phase: group interviews. Report prepared by Scottish Health Feedback for the Greater Glasgow Health Board, 1992.

32. Powney J. Structured eavesdropping. Research Intelligence. *Journal of the British Educational Research Foundation* 1988; **28**: 3–4.

33. MacDougall C & Baum F. The devil's advocate: a strategy to avoid groupthink and stimulate discussion in focus groups. *Qualitative Health Research* 1997; **7**: 532–541.

34. Morgan D & Kreguer R. *The Focus Group Kit,* vols. 1–6. SAGE, London, 1997.

35. Kitzinger J. Audience understanding AIDS: a discussion of methods. *Sociology of Health and Illness* 1990; **12**: 319–335.

36. Myers G & Macnaghten P. Can focus groups be analyzed as talk? In: Barbour R & Kitzinger J, eds. *Developing Focus Group Research: Politics, Theory and Practice.* SAGE, London, 1999.

37. Kitzinger J & Farquhar C. The analytical potential of 'sensitive moments' in focus group discussions. In: Barbour R & Kitzinger J, eds. *Developing Focus Group Research: Politics, Theory and Practice.* SAGE, London, 1999.

38. Waterton C & Wynne B. Can focus groups access community views? In: Barbour R & Kitzinger J. *Developing Focus Group Research: Politics, Theory and Practice.* SAGE, London, 1999.

CHAPTER 4

Observational methods

Catherine Pope, Nicholas Mays

Chapters 2 and 3 described methods that allow researchers to collect data largely based on what people say. Interviewees and focus group members report their beliefs and attitudes, and may also talk about their actions and behaviour. One benefit of these methods is that they provide a relatively quick way of gathering this sort of information, but we cannot be sure that what people say they do is what they actually do [1,2]. Observational methods go some way towards addressing this problem – instead of asking questions about behaviour, the researcher systematically watches people and events to observe everyday behaviours and relationships. As a result, observation is particularly appropriate for studying how organisations work, the roles played by different staff and the interaction between staff and clients.

Observation is the building block of the natural sciences: the biologist observes the development of cell structures and the chemist observes chemical reactions. Observational studies of populations or communities are used in epidemiology to look for patterns in the incidence of disease. Research in clinical and experimental psychology relies on observation, as does the monitoring of a patient in a hospital bed. Qualitative research uses systematic, detailed observation of behaviour and talk. One of the crucial differences between this type of observation and that conducted in the natural sciences is that in the social world those we observe can use language to describe, reflect on, and argue about what they are doing. This shared understanding of the social world between participants and researchers makes this type of social science research very different from the observation of laboratory rats or electrons. Unlike the natural sciences, qualitative observation normally aspires to be *naturalistic* in that people are studied in situ with as little interference by the researcher as is feasible and ethical [3].

Uses of observational methods in health research

Observational methods are often viewed as synonymous with *ethnography*, an approach to research derived from the techniques used by anthropologists to study small-scale societies and different cultures (see below), though ethnographers often use other methods as well. Early anthropologists would live in these societies and cultures for long periods of time, attempting to document behaviours and learn about language, belief systems and social structures. In the 1920s, researchers connected with the so-called Chicago School of sociology began to use ethnographic methods to study the urban environment with which they were familiar, and to systematically observe the lives of different, often marginal or deviant social groups such as gamblers, drug addicts and jazz musicians. Early examples of the use of observational methods in health research include Roth's pioneering study of a TB sanatorium in which he developed the concept of the 'patient career' – a series of stages that the patient passes through during treatment – and the idea of 'timetables' that structure the treatment process for both patients and staff [4]. In the United Kingdom, there have been a number of observational studies of accident and emergency (A and E) departments. Jeffery [5] documented the categorisation by staff of patients into the 'good' and the 'rubbish', the latter consisting of drunks, vagrants, para-suicides and other patients who, because of the conflicting demands and pressures on staff, were seen as inappropriate attenders at A and E. Dingwall and Murray [6] developed and extended this model using observation and interviews to examine how children were managed in A and E. In another study, Hughes [7] observed reception clerks' use of discretion when prioritising and categorising A and E attenders. These studies provide clear insights as to how and why patients are managed as they are in such settings. The behaviour of staff in categorising and labelling patients was so embedded in the organisational culture that only an outsider would have considered it noteworthy. It is unlikely that interviews alone would have been able to uncover the patient typologies used by the staff and the different patterns of care they provoked.

Observational research has been used to develop explanations for relationships or associations found in quantitative work. Bloor's [8] observational study of ear, nose and throat (ENT) surgeons was designed to complement a statistical analysis of variations between areas and surgeons in rates of childhood tonsillectomy. Bloor systematically observed how surgeons made their decisions to operate and discovered that individual doctors had different 'rules of thumb' for deciding whether or not to intervene. While one surgeon might take clinical signs as the chief indication for surgery, another might be prepared to operate in the absence of such indications at the time of consultation if there was evidence that repeated episodes of tonsillitis were affecting a child's education.

Hughes and Griffiths [9] observed cardiac catheterisation clinics and neurological admissions conferences to explore how decisions about treatment priorities between individual patients were made when resources were constrained. They showed that patient selection differed dramatically between the two specialties and suggested that this could be explained by the way rationing decisions were made in each. They showed that in cardiology, decisions tended be framed around the idea of poor prognosis or unsuitability of the patient – 'ruling out' – whereas in neurology, greater weight tended to be placed on 'ruling in' – identifying factors that might make an individual patient especially deserving of help. These analyses begin to explain why different types of patients come to be treated and might be helpful in designing more explicit priority-setting systems in future.

Observational methods have been used to look at the everyday work of health professionals [10–13], and other members of the health care team – for example, the clerks who deal with inpatient waiting lists [14]. There is also a growing body of even more explicitly policy-oriented observational research. Strong and Robinson's [15] analysis of the introduction of general management in the NHS in the mid-1980s involved the researchers sitting in on management meetings as well as conducting lengthy interviews with those involved in the transition to the new-look NHS. Observational methods were subsequently used to look at the relative importance of relations built on trust versus more adversarial relationships in negotiating effective contracts for health services in the NHS internal market of the first half of the 1990s [16]. It is now common in qualitative policy evaluations to use observation to corroborate or nuance accounts given by interviewees (see Chapter 10 on case studies). For example, interviews may reveal a particular approach to decision making in a health services organisation which can then be studied more narrowly, but directly, by observing how specific decisions are taken.

Access to the field and research roles

The first task in observational research is choosing and gaining access to the setting or 'field'. Occasionally, access to the setting leads to opportunistic research – Roth [4] happened to have TB when he conducted his research on life in a TB hospital – but few researchers have it this easy (or difficult). Most have to decide on the type of setting they are interested in and negotiate access. The choice of setting is typically purposive; the idea is not to choose a setting to generalise to a whole population (as would be the case in a statistical sample), but to select a group or setting that is likely to demonstrate salient features and events or categories of behaviour relevant to the research question. Hughes and Griffiths deliberately selected the very different settings of a neurology and a cardiology clinic as the basis for their research on micro-level rationing to allow them to look at two contrasting areas of clinical practice where significant resource constraints apply.

Access to a setting or group is often negotiated via a 'gatekeeper', someone in a position to allow and, ideally, to facilitate the research. In health care settings, this may involve negotiating with different staff, including doctors, nurses, and managers. The first and principal point of contact is important: this person may be seen to sponsor or support the research and this can affect how the researcher is perceived by the group. This can be problematic, as Atkinson [17] found in his study of haematologists: although he had gained access via a very senior member of staff, he initially encountered hostility and some resistance from more junior staff and had to work hard to be accepted by the group. It can be difficult to develop sufficient rapport and empathy with the group to enable the research to be conducted. The researcher may be expected to reciprocate the favour of having been granted access, perhaps through subtle pressure to produce a broadly positive account. Even without this pressure, it is not uncommon for observers to become embroiled in the life of the setting, to the extent of being asked to assist with clerking patients, running errands, or simply holding a nervous patient's hand. This is not necessarily a bad thing (see below) as long as the researcher is aware that this increases the likelihood of not only empathising with the staff but also perhaps siding with them.

It is important to consider the characteristics of the researcher as well as those of the group or setting, as this too influences the process of data collection: being male or female, young or old, naïve or experienced, can affect the interactions between the researcher and the researched [18–19]. The researcher needs to be accepted by the group but avoid 'going native' (that is becoming so immersed in the group culture that the researcher either loses the ability to stand back and analyse the setting, or finds it extremely difficult or emotionally draining to conclude the data collection.)

The observer may adopt different roles according to the type of setting and to how access was obtained. Some health care settings are semi-public spaces, and it may be possible to adhere closely to the role of detached observer, unobtrusively watching what goes on. However, the presence of an observer, particularly in more private settings, may stimulate modifications in behaviour or action – the so-called Hawthorne effect [20,21] – although this effect seems to reduce over time. Those being observed may also begin to reflect on their activities and question the observer about what they are doing.

The impact of the observer on the setting can be minimised in some cases by participating in the activities taking place while observing them. Sometimes this is done covertly, as in Goffman's research [22] on the asylum where he worked as physical education instructor, or in Rosenhan's study [23] where observers feigned psychiatric symptoms to gain admission to a psychiatric hospital. There are important ethical issues in such research. Covert research roles may be justified in certain circumstances such as researching particularly sensitive topics or difficult-to-access groups. Most research in health care settings is overt, although the extent to which all members of the group need to know about the research may vary. For example, staff and patients (and sometimes staff but not patients) may be aware that observation is taking place, but they may not know the specific research questions or areas of interest. Such research often entails continual, informal negotiation of access and consent, although this may not be practical in all settings [24,25]. In the health field, research ethics committees, accustomed to regulating clinical research, may insist on fully informed consent procedures that can jeopardise the feasibility of certain observational studies by alerting participants and, thereby, altering their behaviour (see Chapter 6 for more on this issue).

Recording observational data

Observational research relies on the researcher acting as the research instrument and documenting the world she or he observes. This requires not only good observational skills, but good memory and clear, detailed and systematic recording. The research role adopted, whether covert or overt, participant or non-participant, can influence the process of recording. Sometimes it is possible to take notes or record information in the setting, at other times this may be impractical or off-putting. Remembering events and conversations is crucial, and is a skill that requires practice. Memory can be aided by the use of jotted notes made where possible during observation (one way of making such notes is to find excuses to leave the setting for a few minutes to write up – frequent trips to the lavatory are often used for this, though, inevitably, any time away means that episodes of activity are missed!).

Some researchers use a structured list of items to observe and make notes about the layout of the setting, the character of each participant, or a specific set of activities. Silverman used such an approach in his study of paediatric cardiology clinics. Having observed ten clinics, he developed a coding form for recording 'disposal' decisions, which covered the factors that appeared, on the basis of these initial observations, to be involved in those decisions – things such as clinical and social factors, and how and when decisions were communicated to patients [26]. Another way of structuring observation is to focus on 'critical incidents' – discrete events or specific contexts – and to describe and document these separately [27].

Initial notes or jottings to record key events, quotes, and impressions serve as a prompt to full fieldnotes that ideally should be written up as soon as possible after the observation period. Fieldnotes provide detailed, highly descriptive accounts of what was observed, a chronology of events, and a description of the people involved, their talk and their behaviour. It is important that concrete descriptions are recorded, and not simply impressions. Accordingly, there are conventions for denoting different types of observation, such as verbatim quotes from conversations, non-verbal behaviour and gestures or spatial representations. In addition, the researcher needs to document his or her personal impressions, feelings and reactions to these observations. These more reflexive data are typically recorded separately in a research diary. Different researchers have different styles of writing – they may prefer writing in the first or third person, and fieldnotes may be constructed as real time accounts (i.e. in the present tense) or retrospective 'end-point' descriptions. Emerson *et al.* [28] provide a more detailed exposition of the various styles and formats that can be used. Suffice to say, the process of writing takes considerable time and is not straightforward.

Fieldnotes provide a written record of observation, but they are only the raw material of the research and do not by themselves provide explanations. The researcher has to sift, decode and make sense of the data to make them meaningful. This analytical process is entwined with the data collection and the writing up, when the researcher is constantly thinking about what he or she has observed. Emerging categories or tentative hypotheses about the data may be tested during the fieldwork; more cases or examples (or contradictory ones), may be sought.

Observational methods and ethnography

Observational techniques are frequently employed in studies that adopt an ethnographic approach. The term *ethnography* (literally, 'the study of the people'), rather confusingly, refers both to the research process (including design and methods) and the product of the research (i.e. the written report) [29]. The premise underlying ethnography is that to understand a group of people, the researcher needs to observe their daily lives, ideally living with them and living like them. Ethnography emphasises the importance of understanding the symbolic world in which people live, seeing things the way they do and grasping the meanings they draw on to make sense of their experiences. This entails prolonged contact with the setting and groups being studied – a process that researchers describe as 'immersion'. Observation is central to this process and can be used exclusively, but more typically, ethnographic research incorporates other methods, such as interviews and uses qualitative and quantitative data, including documents, routine statistics and so on. As a result, it can have much in common with case study research (see Chapter 10) and the two terms are sometimes used interchangeably.

Ethnographers have used observation to examine health beliefs [30], the organisation of health care [7,14], and medical training [31,32]. One ethnography of how diagnoses of terminal illness are communicated to patients used observation of a hospital ward and clinics, as well as informal conversations and formal interviews with patients and staff [33]. Some indication of how well the principal field worker got to know the families involved is that she also attended some of the funerals of patients and interviewed bereaved spouses. The study team used all these data to show that both patients and their doctors colluded in creating 'false optimism' about recovery and that features of the care process (such as a focus on the timetable of treatment) supported this optimism, which many patients later came to regret.

Theorising from observational research

The analysis of observational data is described in more detail in Chapter 7. In essence it entails close reading and rereading of all the fieldnotes, and an iterative process of developing categories, and testing and refining them to develop theories and explanations. Different methodological and theoretical perspectives can influence this process and the way in which observational data are treated. These different stances are complex and hotly debated, and there is insufficient space to describe them in detail here; interested readers may wish to consult further sources [34–36] as well as reading Chapter 7.

Quality in observational studies

The quality of observational studies depends more than most methods on the quality of the researcher. There is a particular responsibility on the researcher to provide detailed descriptions of data collection and analysis. Details about how the research was conducted are crucial to assessing its integrity; for example, enabling the reader to know how much time was spent in the field, the researcher's proximity to the action or behaviour discussed, how typical the events recorded were and whether any attempts were made to verify the observations made (such as observing comparable settings or seeking out other sources of information, such as documents). It may be possible to check the verisimilitude (the appearance of truthfulness) of an observational study against previous research in similar settings or with similar groups, but perhaps the ultimate test for observational research is *congruence* [37]: how far the research provides the necessary instructions or rules that might enable another researcher to enter and 'pass' (i.e. function as an accepted participant) in that setting or group.

One criticism of much contemporary ethnography in health care settings is that it seldom adheres to the original idea of 'immersion' – few researchers are able to live with the group they are studying for a long, indeterminate period. Instead they tend to concentrate on a particular setting (e.g. a ward) or institution for a planned period of time. As Hammersely points out [38], their participation in the setting is also generally part time and there is a danger that such research will fail to take account of wider, systemic institutional change, cyclical patterns of activity and longer term change within the specific organisation. This is a valid point and researchers, therefore, need to ensure that sufficient data are captured and be careful about the assumptions they derive from their periodic and relatively short-term observations. It is important to ensure that the research design maximises the range of behaviours and people observed, incorporating different times of day, days of the week, months and so on, to spend as much time as possible with the group being studied. Some researchers choose to sample random blocks of time, or observe particular aspects of the setting, or particular individuals for a fixed period and then move on – say, observing the clinic from the reception area and then moving to the nurses' station. Others use the findings from their earlier observations to identify particular times or activities that are likely to be more important to observe in greater depth. It is a mistake to think that the observer will necessarily capture 'everything'. Even the presence of several observers or video and audio taping cannot ensure this. The combination of the practicalities of observation, and the inevitable limitations of recall and perception means that it is simply not possible to record everything. Nonetheless, as far as possible, the researcher's task is to document in detail what happened.

Chapter 8 discusses these issues in greater detail as they relate to identifying and ensuring quality in qualitative research in general. Done systematically and carefully, observational studies can reveal and explain important features of life in health care settings that are not accessible in other ways. The very best, like Goffman's classic study of the asylum [22], can generate insightful and enduring concepts that can be applied to other settings and that add immensely to our knowledge of the social world.

Further reading

Hammersley M & Atkinson P. *Ethnography: Principles in Practice*, 2nd edn. Routledge, London, 1995.

References

1. Silverman D. *Interpreting Qualitative Data*. SAGE, London, 1994.
2. Heritage J. *Garfinkel and Ethnomethodology*. Polity, Cambridge, 1984.

3. Blumer H. *Symbolic Interactionism.* Prentice Hall, Engelwood Cliffs, NJ, 1969.
4. Roth J. *Timetables.* Bobbs-Merrill, NewYork, 1963.
5. Jeffery R. Normal rubbish: deviant patients in casualty departments. *Sociology of Health and Illness* 1979; **1**: 90–108.
6. Dingwall R & Murray T. Categorisation in accident departments: 'good' patients, 'bad' patients and children. *Sociology of Health and Illness* 1983; **5**: 127–148.
7. Hughes D. Paper and people: the work of the casualty reception clerk. *Sociology of Health and Illness* 1989; **11**: 382–408.
8. Bloor M. Bishop Berkeley and the adenotonsillectomy enigma: an exploration of the social construction of medical disposals. *Sociology* 1976; **10**: 43–61.
9. Hughes D & Griffiths L. 'Ruling in' and 'ruling out': two approaches to the microrationing of health care. *Social Science and Medicine* 1997; **44**: 589–599.
10. Clarke P & Bowling A. Quality of life in long stay institutions for the elderly: an observational study of long stay hospital and nursing home care. *Social Science and Medicine* 1990; **30**: 1201–1210.
11. Fox N. *The Social Meaning of Surgery.* Open University Press, Milton Keynes, 1988.
12. Allen D. The nursing-medical boundary: a negotiated order? *Sociology of Health and Illness* 1997; **19**: 498–520.
13. Smith AF, Goodwin D, Mort M *et al.* Expertise in practice: an ethnographic study exploring acquisition and use of knowledge in anaesthesia. *British Journal of Anaesthesia* 2003; **91**: 319–328.
14. Pope C. Trouble in store: some thoughts on the management of waiting lists. *Sociology of Health and Illness* 1991; **13**: 193–212.
15. Strong P & Robinson J. *The NHS: Under New Management.* Open University Press, Milton Keynes, 1990.
16. Flynn R, Williams G & Pickard S. *Markets and Networks: Contracting in Community Health Services.* Open University Press, Buckingham, 1996.
17. Atkinson P. *Medical Talk and Medical Work.* SAGE, London, 1995.
18. Warren C & Rasmussen P. Sex and gender in field research. *Urban Life* 1977; **6**: 349–369.
19. Ostrander S. 'Surely you're not just in this to be helpful': access, rapport, and interviews in three studies of elites. In: Hertz R & Imber J, eds. *Studying Elites Using Qualitative Methods.* SAGE, London, 1995.
20. Roethlisberger FJ & Dickson WJ. *Management and the Worker.* Harvard University Press, Cambridge, MA, 1939.
21. Holden J & Bower P. How does misuse of the term 'Hawthorne effect' affect the interpretation of research outcomes? (Questions and Answers) *Journal of Health Services Research and Policy* 1998; **3**: 192.

22. Goffman E. *Asylums: Essays on the Social Situation of Mental Patients and Other Inmates.* Penguin, Harmondsworth, 1961.
23. Rosenhan DL. On being sane in insane places. *Science* 1973; **179**: 250–258.
24. Dingwall R. Ethics and ethnography. *Sociological Review* 1980; **28**: 871–891.
25. Goodwin D, Pope C, Mort M *et al.* Ethics and ethnography: an experiential account. *Qualitative Health Research,* 2003; **13**: 567–577.
26. Silverman D. The child as a social object: Down's Syndrome children in a paediatric cardiology clinic. *Sociology of Health and Illness* 1989; **3**: 254–274.
27. Erlandson D, Harris E, Skipper B *et al. Doing Naturalistic Inquiry: A Guide to Methods.* SAGE, Newbury Park, CA, 1993.
28. Emerson R, Fretz R & Shaw L. *Writing Ethnographic Fieldnotes.* University of Chicago Press, Chicago, 1995.
29. Savage J. Ethnography and health care. *British Medical Journal* 2000: **321**: 1400–1402.
30. Davidson C, Davey Smith G & Frankel S. Lay epidemiology and the prevention paradox: the implications of coronary candidacy for health education. *Sociology of Health and Illness* 1991; **13**: 1–19.
31. Atkinson PA. *The Clinical Experience,* 2nd edn. Ashgate, Aldershot, 1997.
32. Sinclair S. *Making Doctors.* Berg, Oxford, 1997.
33. The A, Hak T, Koëter G *et al.* Collusion in doctor-patient communication about imminent death: an ethnographic study. *British Medical Journal* 2000; **321**: 1376–1381
34. Van Maanan J. *Tales of the Field: On Writing Ethnography.* University of Chicago Press, Chicago, 1988.
35. Hammersley M. *The Dilemma of Qualitative Method: Herbert Blumer and the Chicago Tradition.* Routledge, London, 1989.
36. Feldman M. *Strategies for Interpreting Qualitative Data. Qualitative Research Methods 33.* SAGE, Newbury Park, CA, 1995.
37. Fielding N. *Researching Social Life.* SAGE, London, 1993.
38. Hammersley M. Ethnography: problems and prospects. Paper presented to the Qualitative Research Methodology Seminar Series, School of Nursing and Midwifery and the School of Education, University of Southampton (sponsored by the ESRC National Centre for Research Methods) 20 January 2005.

CHAPTER 5

Conversation analysis

Sarah Collins, Nicky Britten

Communication between patients and health care professionals both constitutes and reflects the process of health care. Conversation analysis (hereafter CA) provides a means of studying the precise ways in which, through communication in health care consultations, patients' concerns are presented and addressed, symptoms are described and understood, diagnoses are offered and accepted, and treatment options are negotiated and decided on [1–3]. As mentioned earlier in Chapter 3, CA can also be used to analyse focus groups, particularly when these comprise 'naturally occurring' groups such as people who work together.

CA is founded on the premise that social interaction is constructed turn by turn. Through their successive spoken and non-verbal actions, people carry out such everyday activities as making a request, giving advice or registering a complaint. In a health care consultation, patients and professionals enact a host of activities relevant to a patient's care. By communicating in a turn-taking system, they display their own, and shape one another's, interpretations of the activities. Furthermore, in the observable details of their interactions, participants' interpretations are made available to the researcher.

Answering questions of practical and everyday relevance

The sociologist, Harvey Sacks [4], was the first to use CA in a health care setting. A suicide prevention call centre for an emergency psychiatric service contacted Sacks with a practical problem – how to get callers to give their name in a situation fraught with sensitivities. Sacks explored the problem and its solutions through studying the details, design and sequencing of the opening turns of calls made to the centre. Sacks focused his investigation on sequential considerations and on the turn-taking system. When the answerers of calls to the emergency psychiatric service ask, in the opening turn, 'What is your name?', the caller may (in this delicate situation) not freely offer it; but instead ask 'Why?' (perhaps feeling ashamed, or unprepared to divulge this personal information). Or, if the answerer simply says 'Hello' on picking up the phone, the caller may offer a similar greeting in return, proceed to state the reason for calling and bypass the opportunity to give a name. By contrast, if the answerer gives his/her name in the opening greeting, this provides a natural slot for the caller to respond with hers/his. But if, for example, the person calling asks the answerer to repeat his/her opening line (perhaps they didn't hear it) the caller may never give a name. Thus, through the exploration of these alternatives and their consequences, the opening line by the service-provider can be seen to influence the response the caller supplies. Such observations of the design of opening exchanges can be extended to other forms of social and institutional encounter. They also encourage investigation of other circumstances that dictate how, where and whether people reveal information that may be crucial, for example, to their effective care.

The principles of conversation analysis

Sacks' study demonstrates the three fundamental principles of CA:

1 Spoken utterances and non-verbal behaviour perform social actions that are bound up with the broader activities of an encounter (e.g. finding out a person's name).
2 Spoken and non-verbal actions embody participants' turns at talk, and these turns are connected in sequences, such that what one participant says and does is generated by, and dependent upon, what the other participant says and does (e.g. how the caller responds to the greeting given by the person she/he called).
3 These turn and sequence designs recur across instances and exhibit stable patterns (e.g. the design of the opening line given out to several callers will bring a particular, recurring response in turn).

Conducting a CA study in a health care setting

A CA researcher begins by making recordings of naturally occurring interactions between two or more people. In a health care setting, the recording is most commonly (but not exclusively) of face-to-face consultations in the clinic or surgery.

The number and range of consultations recorded depend on the research aims and on the resources available; but generally speaking, a CA study will collect multiple instances (perhaps 20, perhaps 200) of a type of consultation, between one or more types of patient and health professional. This enables recurring communication features, turn designs and sequential patterns (e.g. beyond an individual health professional's communicative style and across different types of consultation) and their variations to be identified.

Decisions also need to be made about how to record. Video-recording enables gestures and body postures to be noted. However, it also raises practical and ethical questions concerning the obtrusiveness of the camera and participants' consent (see Chapter 6).

The first step in the process of analysis is repeated viewing and listening to the recordings. This enables the researcher to become familiar with the raw data, to identify features of note and to collect examples of recurring patterns. This process of listening and viewing is assisted by making a transcript that includes features such as loudness, pace, timed intervals in the talk, and details of gaze direction and posture (see description of some CA notation in Box 5.1).

Initial observations might concern, for example, the opening line of the consultation, the sequence of talk that delivers diagnostic

---

Box 5.1 Selected features of the CA transcription notation system

[ ]	Brackets mark the point at which an ongoing utterance is joined by another and where overlap ends
=	Equals signs show that one utterance continues directly from a prior utterance
:	A colon indicates extension of the sound or syllable it follows
°°	Degree signs denote talk that is quieter than the talk surrounding it
hhh	Audible aspiration
.hhh	Audible inhalation
> <	Talk delivered at a pace quicker than the surrounding talk
↑ ↓	Marked rise/fall in pitch

Adapted from Jefferson [5].

news, the phrasing of a treatment option, or gestures that invoke the use of a computer in the patient–professional interaction. These observations are then refined through detailed description of turn-taking and sequences, and exploration of their specific interactional consequences. Deviant cases are also investigated. Cases of participants' 'resistance' to a particular activity format (e.g. declining to answer a question, or continuing to talk on a prior topic in the face of a marked shift to a new one) can attest to that activity's characteristic design and help to reveal participants' orientation to it. This analytic process requires close and repeated attention to the actual recordings as well as to the transcripts.

Applications of CA research in health care

In recent years, CA has made significant advances in understanding how health care is delivered by health professionals and received by patients. Much of the progress that has been made is attributable to the principle of comparative analysis. CA research in health care compares 'institutional' communication with everyday conversation [6], to reveal the particular rules and practices that govern health care consultations. The benefits of this comparative approach were illustrated earlier with reference to Sacks [4], and further examples are detailed below.

The following examples illustrate the sorts of health care activities that CA research has investigated: the openings of consultations [7]; doctors' 'commentaries' during physical examination [8]; patients' explanations of their illness [9]; and the co-ordination of talk with non-verbal activities during consultations [10]. Two particular studies help to illustrate the sorts of findings generated by CA and their implications for health care research and practice. One study concerns diagnosis; the other concerns treatment.

Maynard [11] identified the so-called perspective-display series as a means of delivering diagnostic news. Doctors may either present their diagnoses immediately, or they may deliver their diagnoses 'circuitously' through the 'perspective-display series', thereby incorporating the carer's or patient's perspective, through a sequence of three turns:

1 doctor's perspective-display invitation;
2 patient's/carer's reply or assessment; and
3 doctor's report and assessment.

From this schematic representation, it can be observed that this series offers the potential for the doctor to accommodate the patient's/carer's perspective on the situation (turn 2) in the diagnostic report that follows (turn 3). Consider the following extract from Maynard's study (see Box 5.2). The extract comes from a recording of a consultation between a parent and a doctor in a clinic for children who have developmental disabilities. In this consultation, the doctor presents the diagnosis of the child's disability.

Box 5.2 An example of the perspective-display series

```
1   Dr:   What do you see? As- as his (0.5) difficulty.
2         (1.2)
3   Mo:   Mainly his uhm: (1.2) the fact that he
4         doesn't understand everything. (0.6) and
5         also the fact that his speech (0.7) is very
6         hard to understand what he's saying (0.3)
7         lot[s of ti]me
8   Dr:      [ right ]
9         (0.2)
10  Dr:   Do you have any ideas why it is? are you:
11        d[o yo]u? h
12  Mo:    [ No ]
13        (2.1)
14  Dr:   .h okay I (0.2) you know I think we basically
15        (.) in some ways agree with you: (0.6) .hh
16        insofar as we think that (0.3) Dan's main
17        problem (0.4) .h you know does: involve you
18        know language.
19        (0.4)
20  Mo:   Mm hmm
21        (0.3)
22  Dr:   you know both (0.2) you know his- (0.4) being
23        able to understand you know what is said to
24        him (0.4) .h and also certainly also to be
25        able to express:: (1.3) you know his uh his
26        thoughts
27        (1.1)
28  Dr:   .hh uh:m (0.6) .hhh in general his
29        development...
```

The doctor begins by asking the mother how she regards her child's difficulty (line 1). The mother is thus invited to present her perspective on her child's problem. In response (in lines 3–7), she reports that her child's difficulties relate to understanding others and to the unintelligibility of his own speech. The doctor pursues her response by asking the mother for her ideas as to why her child has these difficulties (lines 10–11). The mother replies that she has no idea. The doctor then begins to formulate the clinical diagnosis of the child's problem (lines 14–29) and shows how this diagnosis aligns with the perspective that the mother has presented ('we basically in some ways agree with you...', lines 14–15)). He makes explicit reference to each of the difficulties the mother has identified and reformulates them ('Dan's main problem... does... involve language... both... being able to understand what is said to him and... to be able to express... his thoughts').

This example shows how the doctor's talk creates an environment hospitable to the delivery of difficult news, by inviting and building on the parent's perspective. In this example, the process appears relatively straightforward. But a parent may, in reply to the invitation, take a 'no problem' stance. The use of the 'perspective-display series' offers ways of circumventing this – the clinician may (as in another of Maynard's examples) begin by asking, 'How's Bobby doing', and then, as above, reformulate parts of the parent's reply to introduce a problem diagnosis. This particular delivery format also offers other possibilities – in the third turn, the clinician may upgrade the diagnosis, or, alternatively, in cases where parents appear unreceptive to the diagnosis, retreat from an initial formulation to produce one more acceptable to the parent. Thus, through the 'perspective-display series', clinicians can gradually unfold the diagnosis in alignment with parents' or patients' perspectives. This is a process that the alternative delivery format – straightforward assertion – does not allow.

The second example is Stivers' [12] research on antibiotic prescribing decisions in parents' consultations with their children's doctors. She identifies four ways in which parents resist and shape doctors' treatment recommendations and pressurise doctors to prescribe antibiotics for their children. Two of these, overt requests for antibiotics, and explicit statements of a desire for antibiotics, were relatively uncommon in her data. It was more common for parents to advocate the use of antibiotics indirectly – either by simply inquiring about them, or by mentioning a past experience of them. Here is one

---

Box 5.3 Parental pressure for antibiotics through mention of past experience

```
1   Dr:   So:- Let's take uh listen to 'er chest,
2   Mo:   (Alright),
3         (.)
4   Mo:   Remember she- she:=uhm had something like this:
5         in December?
6   Dr:   Uh huh,
7         (0.5)
8   Gir:  Hhh. = .h
9   Mo:   (n') She was on an antibiotic.
10        (1.0)
11  Dr:   Doo doo. ((to girl))
12  Gir:  Ksh:::::, uh.
13  Dr:   Yeah: Well I think that she probably got:=similar
14        type of thi:ng, ya know [some sort of a secondary-
15  Mo:                          [Mm hm:,
16        .hh uh: respiratory infection in her ches:t, like
17        uh bronchitis an'-
```

---

example (see Box 5.3). The parent has already presented the child's problem, and in line 1, the doctor begins the physical examination.

The mother's assertion (lines 4–5, 9) that her daughter had a similar problem before that was treated with antibiotics conveys her position that this present illness is similar and thus requires the same treatment. By asserting this at the onset of physical examination, the mother presents this information as potentially affecting the doctor's treatment recommendation. The doctor initially does not respond, but examines the girl (lines 10–12). He follows this by agreeing with the mother ('yeah') and suggesting that this illness is similar (lines 13–14). The doctor goes on to prescribe antibiotics. The mother has not explicitly requested that antibiotics be prescribed, nor has she stated her preference for them. She has simply offered information. By this indirect and subtle route, the mother's talk influences the prescribing decision the doctor makes.

These two examples show how investigating the details of interaction between patients and health care professionals not only informs understanding of the processes of communication in consultations, but also potentially has consequences for the provision of health care and for professionals' communication practice.

Maynard's [11] research demonstrates a sequential strategy for giving sensitive diagnostic news, by which doctors can enlist the patient's/carer's participation in constructing the diagnosis. A similar resource is found in conversation; but in conversation, the news told in the second turn may then be elaborated by the recipient in the third turn. In health care consultations, the convergence of patient and clinician perspectives is actively managed by the clinician who, in the third turn in the sequence, always delivers his/her medical diagnosis. Maynard's study illustrates one respect in which patients' participation is closely connected to the ways health professionals organise their talk.

Stivers [12] shows that the resources on which patients draw to exert their influence can be subtle. She found that when parents communicate pressure for antibiotics, doctors may prescribe them even when their appropriateness is questionable. Her research highlights the intricacies of communication in consultations – in particular, the 'problematic convergence' between parent participation and antibiotic prescribing, and the difficulties for doctors who must 'encourage and maintain participation whilst simultaneously not giving in to pressure to prescribe inappropriately'.

CA research on everyday conversation has shown that a pause following a question may indicate a disagreement or some other resistance to respond on the part of the answerer. In health care consultations, a pause may indicate resistance on the patient's part to the proposal being offered. On the other hand, Stivers [13] shows how particular treatment recommendation formats are less likely to meet with patients' resistance than are others. Her findings are significant, given the limited communication resources patients have available, and the tendency for communication details to be overlooked in health care research and practice.

Conclusion

This chapter has introduced the basic principles of CA and demonstrated how these have been applied in health care research. The examples given illustrate the variety of CA studies and their contribution to understanding the details of health care communication and the various activities it serves. CA provides a means of investigating patient–professional interaction directly and relatively naturalistically (see Chapter 1 for a discussion of naturalism in qualitative research). It does not rely on retrospective accounts, and, as the researcher is not physically present, the raw data are not structured by the researcher at the point of creation except in the initial selection of which interaction to study. Thus, it offers something distinct from other qualitative methods such as the semi-structured interview, focus group, or observation where the impact of the researcher is more obvious. As a result, CA can provide a strong complement when combined with these other methods.

CA is a method that carefully and systematically describes the details of social interaction, for example, between patients, carers and health professionals. This is a demanding task. Thus, CA is not to be undertaken lightly (and training is offered at centres in the United Kingdom and abroad). But it does offer a wealth of insights into the organisation of communication in consultations, into the workings of health care, and into the experiences of patients and health professionals.

Further reading

ten Have P. *Doing Conversation Analysis: A Practical Guide.* SAGE, London, 1999.

References

1. Drew P, Chatwin J & Collins S. Conversation analysis: a method for research in health care professional-patient interaction. *Health Expectations* 2001; **4/1**: 58–71.
2. Peräkylä A. Conversation analysis: a new model of research in doctor-patient communication. *Journal of the Royal Society of Medicine,* 1997; **90**: 205–208.
3. Levinson SC. *Pragmatics.* Cambridge University Press, Cambridge, 1983.
4. Sacks H. *Lectures on Conversation,* Edited by Jefferson G, vols. I and II. Blackwell Publishing, Oxford, 1992.
5. Jefferson G. Transcript notation. In: Atkinson JM & Heritage J, eds. *Structures of Social Action: Studies in Conversation Analysis.* Cambridge University Press, Cambridge, 1984: ix–xvi.
6. Drew P & Heritage J, eds. *Talk at Work: Interaction in Institutional Settings.* Cambridge University Press, Cambridge, 1992.
7. Gafaranga J & Britten N. 'Fire away': the opening sequence in general practice consultations. *Family Practice* 2003; **20**: 242–247.

8. Heritage J & Stivers T. Online commentary in acute medical visits: a method of shaping patient expectations. *Social Science and Medicine* 1999; **49**: 1501–1517.

9. Gill VT. Doing attributions in medical interaction: patients' explanations for illness and physicians' responses. *Social Psychology Quarterly,* 1998; **61**: 342–360.

10. Heath C. *Body Movement and Speech in Medical Interaction.* Cambridge University Press, Cambridge, 1986.

11. Maynard DW. On clinicians co-implicating recipients' perspective in the delivery of diagnostic news. In: Drew & Heritage J, eds. *Talk at Work: Interaction in Institutional Settings.* Cambridge University Press, Cambridge, 1992: 331–358.

12. Stivers T. Participating in decisions about treatment: overt parent pressure for antibiotic medication in pediatric encounters. *Social Science and Medicine* 2002; **54**: 1111–1130.

13. Stivers T. Non-antibiotic treatment recommendations: delivery formats and implications for parent resistance. *Social Science and Medicine* 2005; **60**: 949–964.

CHAPTER 6
Ethical issues

Dawn Goodwin

This chapter explores three ethical issues that are particularly important when undertaking qualitative research: anonymity, confidentiality and informed consent. Qualitative researchers routinely give research participants assurances about anonymity, yet in practice, complete anonymity may be difficult to achieve. It is, therefore, necessary to rethink the level of anonymity that can be attained and how to accomplish this. Similarly, participants may be advised that any information they disclose will remain confidential, although in qualitative research, in contrast to quantitative research, individual respondents' responses – often their exact words – are reproduced. Given this, what does maintaining confidentiality mean? Finally, informed consent has been seen as central to ethical research conduct, but again, how 'informed' can informed consent be? How is informed consent achieved in a qualitative study that evolves as it progresses, in which the significance of information may only become clear as the study develops?

Anonymity

At the beginning of a research project, changing the names of participants and obscuring the location of the research may seem a straightforward means of protecting the identity of research participants [1]. However, in qualitative research the level of detail necessary to support and situate research claims, the use of a single or small number of settings and the relatively small number of participants involved, frequently complicate simple anonymisation. Punch has argued that as many institutions and public figures are almost impossible to disguise, their cooperation in research may incur a certain measure of exposure. The tendency of researchers to choose research locations close to their academic institution can easily undermine the use of pseudonyms for organisations and individuals [2]. These observations apply to research in health care settings. For example, the study of the hospital near the researcher's workplace, or of a group of specialist practitioners may be easily deduced by an inquisitive reader of a report or paper.

Richards and Schwartz [3] argue that problems of anonymity permeate every level of research. Interview transcripts contain multiple clues to a person's identity – their name, employment details, place of residence and events that have occurred in their communities. This may seem an obvious point to mention, and perhaps superfluous if anonymity is only necessary in published accounts, but the anonymity of participants in the early stages of research becomes significant when conducting team research. In health care, particularly, it may be useful to have 'insiders' as co-researchers as members of the community being studied can ease problems of access; they are familiar with the demands of a clinical environment; understand the nomenclature; and can be useful in elucidating points of clinical understanding. Here, assurances of anonymity may alleviate a colleague's potential uneasiness at being 'spied' [4] upon. When the researcher is so familiar with the environment, however, a simple change of name is insufficient to obscure the participant's identity. In some cases, so many details would have to be changed as to make the data senseless. Richards and Schwartz point out that participants will often be known to the person carrying out the transcription, which again is worth considering if using a local transcription service or perhaps even the departmental secretary for this task. Even after processes of anonymisation are applied, quotations, speech mannerisms and context may provide enough information to identify participants, and it is not always easy for the researcher to predict which data could lead to identification [3].

It seems inevitable that when a small number of participants are recruited from one research location, any association of practitioners with the researcher could suggest that they participated in the research. Furthermore, when the research necessarily features the circumstances and events that have given meaning to an individual's life, and that make it different from other lives (e.g. in life history and narrative accounts), identities are not so easily concealed by pseudonyms. All these factors make it difficult to preserve anonymity and have led some [5] to question whether the standard ethical expectations of complete anonymity and confidentiality are appropriate or even feasible for all forms of research.

So, before making commitments of anonymity to research participants there needs to be some consideration of the level of anonymity that can be achieved. This means asking questions about the research such as: How can the research location be adequately disguised? Is it sufficiently 'typical' for a pseudonym to be effective, or should the research design be adapted to include more than one location? Even a short period of comparative data collection at an additional site may help to mask the location being described, as well as the identity of the individuals who generated the data. When it comes to the participants, it may be necessary to consider whether anonymity during the data collection and analysis is needed, and whether this is feasible given that a pseudonym is often insufficient. It may be possible to negotiate disclosure of information and identities with those involved in the research, but sometimes hard decisions may need to be made about what not to report if doing so would compromise the anonymity of participants in ways that could be harmful to them.

Confidentiality

It has been argued that the assurance of confidentiality is the major safeguard against the invasion of privacy through research [2]. However, it is first necessary to question what confidentiality means in qualitative research. As Richards and Schwartz [3] point out, the term 'confidentiality' has different meanings for health care practitioners and researchers. For health care practitioners, confidentiality requires that no personal information is passed on except in exceptional circumstances, but for researchers 'the duty of confidentiality is less clear' [3: 138]. There is a danger in conflating confidentiality and anonymity. To keep something confidential is to keep it private [6]. Thus, while the use of pseudonyms may protect the identity of participants, it does not necessarily mean that what they say will be kept private. It is essential that the researcher is clear at the outset as to what confidentiality means in the context of qualitative research. This involves explaining the kinds of output that might be expected from the study. It may help to clarify the limits to confidentiality – for example, the researcher may be able to confirm that remarks made by a nurse are not reported to his/her colleague or manager who is also a respondent, but cannot guarantee that (suitably anonymised) verbatim quotes will not appear in a final report. Many researchers provide opportunities for participants to see and often, to approve, the data at different stages – for example, by allowing them opportunities to see transcripts and excerpts destined to be used in final reports. This can help to avoid surprise and discontent when participants' 'confidential' comments find their way into research publications, particularly for respondents who are unfamiliar with qualitative research.

One frequent difficulty encountered in qualitative research is that, even when the researcher is openly recording data, such as in interviews, participants may still choose to confide in the researcher, prefacing their disclosure with remarks such as, 'just between ourselves', or they may request the researcher to 'switch the tape recorder off' before they continue [4]. Evidently, the participant wants the researcher to be informed, but for that information to remain private. Burgess' approach to these situations was that although the information could not be used directly such 'data' could inform the researcher's understanding of other situations – situations that could be quoted. A similar problem arises in observational and documentary research when the researcher may have access to documents marked 'confidential'. Once again, whilst these documents may inform the analysis they cannot be directly quoted or referenced [4].

More ambiguous still, are those occasions when the researcher is less obviously 'on duty'. For example, during an observational study of health care work, there may be opportunities to interact with practitioners in less formal settings during meal breaks or social occasions. Incidental conversations may be seen by the participants as the lubrication between research events rather than as part of the research itself. How to handle information garnered informally in this way is a frequent concern in ethnographic research [7]. Dingwall [8] recalls the difficulties incurred when participants realised that data collection entailed recording informal 'backstage' events as well as behaviour in more formal settings. Participants found it difficult to link events and behaviour in the informal sphere with the announced theme of the research. For Dingwall, the issue was 'the morality of using unguarded statements and ... the potential for exploitative relationships' [8: 882]. These tensions are particularly acute in ethnographic research as participants may forget that research is taking place once they come to know the ethnographer as a person [7]. Ethnographers can exacerbate this tension by actively building rapport with participants, in an attempt to minimize reactivity [7] or the Hawthorne effect. This clearly limits confidentiality in the sense of maintaining privacy. In building rapport the researcher may be seen as an ally when engaged in examining the workings of the profession or community, but 'allies are expected to keep secrets and respect proprietary boundaries between public and private', [9: 322] whereas researchers may want to expose these very secrets and boundaries.

Box 6.1 describes a situation where confidentiality was problematic, despite the researcher openly making fieldnotes. This incident prompted deliberations on where to draw the boundaries of confidentiality. These types of decisions are not exceptional but are common to all qualitative research, and they are faced not only at the beginning of research projects but throughout. They are examples of the 'everyday dilemmas' [10] researchers face. When addressing confidentiality in qualitative research the researcher may need to consider differentiating between types of data – that which can be published, that which is circulated between co-researchers, and

---

Box 6.1 Privacy and consent [11]

During observation, the researcher, a former anaesthetic nurse, is openly taking fieldnotes in the operating theatre, watching the anaesthetist at work. Another anaesthetist arrives and the two anaesthetists conduct a conversation that they term 'confidential' in the researcher's presence. The conversation concerns another member of the anaesthetic team who is not present. The questions raised by this episode include: should a 'confidential conversation' be kept private or noted as additional data? Would conveying the content of the conversation to the other researchers breach confidentiality? What were the risks that dissemination of this conversation might harm the individuals involved? Was the researcher being trusted by the participants (her ex-colleagues) to use her discretion and draw a line between public and private?

In the event, the researcher decided not to write notes about the content of the conversation but to record in fieldnotes the questions raised by this event. The situation (but not the content of the conversation) was subsequently discussed by the research team and it was agreed that the conversation should be kept private.

occasionally, that which should be kept in a personal fieldwork journal.

Informed consent

Informed consent 'has become a virtual canon of ethics and research in all fields' [10: 184]. However, this does not mean that informed consent is always straightforward. The main problem for qualitative researchers lies in specifying in advance which data will be collected and how they will be used [4,12]. During interviews, for example, the potential uses of the data are not always clear as the very nature of qualitative research means that unexpected themes can arise during the analysis [3]. For ethnographic research, there is the further problem of carrying out research in naturally occurring settings, and, therefore, having little or no control over who enters the research field and when [7]. As Dingwall recognises, 'so many people are encountered casually that it is impractical to obtain consent on each and every occasion without causing total disruption' [8: 878]. Situations may arise in which there is no opportunity for introductions and where the other participants offer no explanation as to the presence of a researcher [4]. One way of addressing this issue is to be as overt as possible whilst recording data [8]. Although far from foolproof (as Box 6.1 shows), openly recording fieldnotes enables participants to gauge for themselves what they deem appropriate to have 'on the record'.

However, as Hammersley and Atkinson acknowledge, 'even when operating in an overt manner, ethnographers rarely tell *all* the people they are studying *everything* about the research' [7: 265, original italics]. There are various reasons for this, some of which have been mentioned above: initially the research design may deliberately lack specificity; it is often hard to predict in advance precisely which data will become significant; and it may not be possible or appropriate to interrupt the working routines of the research setting. All of these factors contribute to the lack of opportunities to convey details of the research to participants. But even when the research questions and strategy have been clarified, there is still the risk of affecting participants' behaviour by explaining exactly what will be studied [7]. Further, to minimize disruption and remain on good terms with the participant, the researcher may withhold her/his own opinions or agree with the participant's views [7,8]. As Dingwall grants, some level of 'impression management' is always necessary [8].

In health care research, an additional problem is encountered by those researchers who are also health practitioners. When researching in health care settings, observing practice, or talking about services, these researchers may face the additional dilemma of whether and how to intervene should they witness less than optimal attitudes or practices [8] (see example in Box 6.2). Field [13] acknowledges the difficulty for a researcher who is also a member of the community being studied, to step back and observe the setting from a research perspective. She recognises that 'Nurses do not find it easy to sit in a corner and do nothing, particularly in an area that is busy and one they know well' [13: 94]. This difficulty may be exacerbated when colleagues or patients, acting as research participants, know the researcher as a practitioner and do not distinguish between the two roles. The patient may expect that the researcher will not allow anything untoward to occur [13]. In addition, if the researcher only observes, she/he may feel implicated in any poor practice observed.

The purpose of outlining these circumstances and obstacles is not to diminish informed consent as a means of achieving ethical research practice, rather, by appreciating such practical constraints and contingencies the aim is to alert the researcher to the fact that obtaining informed consent in qualitative research cannot be accomplished by the mechanistic production of a consent form signed at the outset of the research [10,12]. 'Informed consent, in its fullest interpretation, means openness and disclosure with participants, and models of research that are collaborative' [10: 190]. Achieving this demands continuous negotiation of the terms of agreement as the study evolves [3,12]. The salient point is that obtaining informed consent in qualitative research is not a once and for always action.

Box 6.2 Practitioner as researcher dilemmas [11]

During an observation session the researcher, who is a registered nurse, notices that the patient's blood pressure had fallen and the fluid infusion had run out. The end of the anaesthetic infusion was imminent. Should the researcher still act as a nurse by alerting the anaesthetist? Does the presence of other patient advocates (nurses and anaesthetists) absolve the researcher of the responsibilities of a nurse?

It may be that for participants whose role in the research is fleeting and transitory, a single brief and honest introduction, outlining the research questions, the data collection strategy, and the overall objectives of the research, is sufficient; whereas for those participants whose engagement in the study is prolonged, who have contributed significantly towards the study's progress, repeated discussions, presentations and progress reports may be necessary both to inform participants adequately, and to secure their continued interest in the success of the study.

Ethical practice

This chapter has discussed the three key ethical issues in conducting qualitative research. Some ethical issues can be anticipated and the study designed accordingly, but many 'everyday dilemmas' [10] will develop unpredictably during the course of the research. These, Punch notes, 'often have to be resolved *situationally* and even spontaneously, without the luxury of being able to turn first to consult a more experienced colleague' [2: 84], or indeed to scrutinize the stipulations of codes of ethical practice (e.g. those on the BSA and SRA websites, detailed at the end of this chapter). Many commentators have recognised that whilst it is possible to prescribe a set of abstract ethical principles, the application of these rules and which actions constitute following these rules, may not be particularly clear in the complexity of the field setting [2,4,7]. Accordingly, Fluehr-Lobban suggests that the value of codes of ethical practice is educational rather than adjudicative [10].

The 'emergent' nature of qualitative studies requires that the researcher relinquish a degree of control over aspects such as the places and times of data collection, the themes that become important, and the topics that participants bring to the research. Accepting this means that sometimes it may not be possible or desirable to avoid acting in ways that run contrary to the values expressed in codes of ethical practice [7]. As Hammersley and Atkinson point out, 'values often conflict, and their implications for what is legitimate and illegitimate in particular situations is, potentially at least, always a matter for reasonable dispute' [7: 280]. To recognise that it is often impossible to determine the balance of benefit to risk prior to a research undertaking is to accept that ethics is a process [14]. Accordingly, a review of ethical problems and dilemmas should be at the heart of reflexive research practice [4]. In every sense, qualitative research is thoroughly negotiated, and ethical practice is more a process than an outcome; it cannot be determined only by the researcher, but is accomplished through negotiations with participants in light of the contingencies of doing research in particular settings.

Further reading

British Sociological Association (BSA). *Statement of Ethical Practice.* www.britsoc.org.uk/about/ethic.htm
Social Research Association (SRA). *Ethical Guidelines.* http://www.thesra.org.uk/ethicals.htm
Green J & Thorogood N. Responsibilities, ethics and values (Chapter 3). In: Green J & Thorogood N, eds. *Qualitative Methods for Health Research.* SAGE, London, 2004.

References

1. Fetterman DM. *Ethnography Step by Step.* SAGE, Newbury Park, 1989.
2. Punch M. Politics and ethics in qualitative research. In: Denzin NK & Lincoln YS, eds. *Handbook of Qualitative Research.* SAGE, Thousand Oaks, 1994: 83–97.
3. Richards HM & Schwartz LJ. Ethics of qualitative research: are there special issues for health services research? *Family Practice* 2002; **19**: 135–139.
4. Burgess RG. Grey areas: ethical dilemmas in educational ethnography. In: Burgess RG, ed. *The Ethics of Educational Research.* The Falmer Press, New York, 1989: 60–76.
5. Boman J & Jevne R. Ethical evaluation in qualitative research. *Qualitative Health Research* 2000; **10**(4): 547–554.
6. *Oxford English Dictionary*, 10th edn. Oxford University Press, Oxford, 1999.
7. Hammersley M & Atkinson P. *Ethnography*, 2nd edn. Routledge, London, 1995.
8. Dingwall R. Ethics and ethnography. *Sociological Review* 1980; **28**(4): 871–891.
9. de Laine M. *Ethnography, Theory and Applications in Health Research.* MacLennan and Petty, Sydney, 1997.
10. Fluehr-Lobban C. Ethics. In: Bernard HR, ed. *Handbook of Methods in Cultural Anthropology.* AltaMira, Walnut Creek, 1998: 173–202.
11. Goodwin D, Pope C, Mort M & Smith A. Ethics and ethnography: an experiential account. *Qualitative Health Research* 2003; **13**(4): 567–577.

12. Hoeyer K, Dahlager L & Lynoe N. Conflicting notions of research ethics: the mutually challenging traditions of social scientists and medical researchers. *Social Science and Medicine* 2005; **61**: 1741–1749.
13. Field, PA. Doing fieldwork in your own culture. In: Morse JM, ed. *Qualitative Nursing Research: A Contemporary Dialogue*, Revised edition. SAGE, Newbury Park, 1991: 91–104.
14. Parnis D, Du Mont J & Gombay B. Cooperation or co-optation? Assessing the methodological benefits and barriers involved in conducting qualitative research through medical institutional settings. *Qualitative Health Research* 2005; **15**(5): 686–697.

CHAPTER 7

Analysing qualitative data

Catherine Pope, Sue Ziebland, Nicholas Mays

The nature and scale of qualitative data

There is a widely held perception that qualitative research is small scale. As it tends to involve smaller numbers of subjects or settings than quantitative research, it is assumed, incorrectly, that it generates fewer data than quantitative research. In fact, qualitative research can produce vast amounts of data. As Chapters 2–5 have suggested, a range of different types of data may be collected during a qualitative study. These may include observational notes, interview and focus group transcripts and documentary material, as well as the researcher's own records of ongoing analytical ideas, research questions, and the field diary, which provides a chronology of the events witnessed and the progress of the research. Each of these different types of data can be substantial. A transcript of a single qualitative interview generates anything between 20 and 40 single-spaced pages of text, and it does not take long for a collection of fieldnotes and documentary materials related to observations of one or two settings to fill a filing cabinet drawer.

Data preparation

Verbatim notes or audio/video tapes of face-to-face interviews or focus groups are transcribed to provide a record of what was said. The preparation of transcribed material will depend on the level of analysis being undertaken, but even if only sections of the data are intended for analysis, the preservation of the original tapes or documents is recommended. Transcribing is time consuming. Each hour of material can take six or seven hours to transcribe depending on the quality of the tape and the depth of information required. For this reason many researchers outsource transcription to commercial or other secretarial services. However, even when using such services, the researcher needs to carefully check each transcript against the original recording and this too can be a lengthy process. Supplying the transcriber with a list of medical and other terms that are likely to appear in the tapes will be helpful, as will clear examples of the style of transcription you prefer. If you plan to use computer software (see below) for analysing the data, do not use different fonts (e.g. italics) to indicate which participant is speaking, because they will be lost when files are converted into text formats.

Conversation analysis of audio-taped material requires even more detailed annotation of a wide range of features of the talk studied, and some of the conventions for annotating transcripts for this purpose are described in Chapter 5, Box5.1. Even when the research is not concerned with analysing talk in this depth it is still important that the data provide an accurate record of what was said and done. The contribution of sighs, laughs and lengthy pauses should not be underestimated when analysing talk, and, as a minimum, these should be noted in the transcription. Transcription can be thought of as a research act because the level and detail of the transcription affects the type of analysis that can be undertaken. Consider, for example, how the inclusion or exclusion of instances of repetition, 'ums' and 'ers', and the record and timing of laughter, crying or pauses can affect the interpretation of speech [1].

Notes made during or immediately after observational work have to be turned into detailed descriptive accounts of the hours spent watching and listening, and taking part in, events, interactions and conversations. This writing process typically requires an extended block of time ideally away from the research setting, but as close as possible to the time when the observation was done.

Whether using interviews or observation, the maintenance of meticulous records is vital – these are the raw data of the research. National qualitative data archives in Britain [2] and the archives of illness narratives produced by qualitative projects such as DIPEx (Personal Experiences of Health and Illness – see www.dipex.org) have made secondary analysis of qualitative data easier, and this means that it is even more important that full records of qualitative studies are kept to allow the possibility of future analysis. It is also important to find ways of filing and storing the data that facilitate retrieval and getting to know the data. Simple techniques like standardised file formats and layouts, along with clear file labelling enable speedy access to data. It is also worth keeping a record of the different types of data collected and their location in the filing or archiving system used.

The relationship between data and analysis

Transcripts and fieldnotes provide a descriptive record, but they cannot provide explanations. The researcher has to make sense of the data by sifting and interpreting them. In most qualitative research the analytical process begins during the data collection phase as the data already gathered are analysed and feed into, or shape, the ongoing data collection. This sequential [3] or interim analysis [4] (see Figure 7.1) allows the researcher to check and interpret the data she/he is collecting continually and to develop hypotheses for subsequent investigation in further data collection. Compared with quantitative methods, this has the advantage of allowing the researcher to go back and refine questions and to pursue emerging avenues of inquiry in further depth. Crucially, it also enables the researcher to seek out deviant or negative cases; that is, examples of talk or events that run counter to the emerging propositions or hypotheses, to refine the argument and interpretation. This type of analysis is almost inevitable in qualitative research; because the researcher is 'in the field' collecting the data, it is impossible not to start thinking about what is being heard and seen.

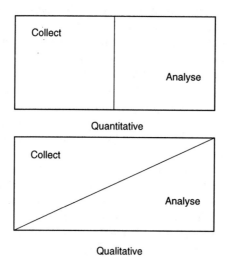

Figure 7.1 Models of the research process.

Counting and qualitative data

Qualitative (i.e. textual) data can be analysed quantitatively. Quantitative content analysis uses an unambiguous, predefined coding system and produces counts or frequencies that may be tabulated and analysed using standard statistical techniques. This approach is often used in media and mass communications studies. In general, qualitative research does not seek to quantify data, although simple counts can be useful in qualitative studies. One example of this approach is Silverman's research on communication in clinics [5]. This quantified features such as consultation length and the patient's use of questions, and combined this information with the qualitative analysis to confirm a series of propositions about the differences between private and NHS clinics. Analysis that counts items in the data should be seen as distinct from qualitative analyses in which the data are preserved in their textual form and interpreted to generate and develop analytical categories and theoretical explanations.

Qualitative researchers usually treat counting with caution. The reasons for this may be illustrated by contrasting the objectives of qualitative research with that of surveys and trials. In a study where everyone within a given population has had an equal chance of being selected to participate (this assumption is the cornerstone of sampling theory) and all respondents have been asked the same questions in the same manner, it is usually helpful to report responses as frequencies and percentages (relative frequencies). Surveys are designed to recruit sufficient numbers to represent the whole population. Trials aim to randomise enough subjects so that significant differences between treatment and control groups can be identified. By contrast, the qualitative methods of interviewing and observation are intended to identify subjective meanings and generate theory (i.e. explanations), which means that data collection will often continue until saturation point has been reached (and no new categories are being contributed by additional data), rather than to be statistically representative. For example, unusual or 'outlier' cases may be actively sought. In a qualitative study where the sample has not been (and often cannot be) selected to be *numerically* representative of the population, and where the interview technique is flexible and responsive, it can be misleading to report relative frequencies. This particularly applies if the questions have not been asked of all respondents, or have not been phrased in the same way or delivered at the same stage in each interview.

Initial steps

Although some analysis is done whilst the data are being collected, there is still much to do once the researcher has left the field. The approach to analysis is influenced by theoretical and methodological perspectives and should relate to the aims of the research. Different styles of research may require differing depths of analysis: the analysis of an interview-based study is likely to be more detailed than the analysis of a small number of interviews carried out as part of a mixed method study that has several components to be analysed. The analysis may seek simply to describe people's views or behaviours, or move beyond this to provide explanations that can take the form of classifications, typologies, patterns, models and theories. Spencer *et al.* liken the analytic structure that underpins this process to scaffolding [6: 213] and suggest that analysis moves iteratively through stages of *data management, description* and *explanation* via a series of 'platforms' from which the researchers can reflect on what they have done and move forward. This process is fluid and, crucially, non-linear; the researcher develops the analysis by moving backwards and forwards between the original data and the emerging interpretations.

Qualitative analysis seeks to develop analytic categories to describe and explain social phenomena. These categories may be derived inductively – that is obtained gradually from the data – or used deductively, either at the beginning or part way through the analysis as a way of approaching the data. There are three broad approaches for taking the analysis forward: *thematic analysis; grounded theory;* and the *framework approach*. These move from the broadly inductive to more deductive approaches, but, in practice, many researchers find that they move between induction and deduction in the same analysis. Sometimes techniques from different analytical approaches are combined to understand the data better.

The first task in the analysis is simply to manage and make sense of the huge array of data collected. This data management stage is broadly similar for each of the three analytical approaches and entails reading and re-reading all the data to identify an initial set of themes or categories. The data are systematically searched for recurring themes and items of interest such as events or views that are unusual, noteworthy or contradictory. For focus group or interview material, this may include searching for particular types of narrative – such as jokes or anecdotes, or types of interaction such as questions, challenges, censorship or changes of mind. In more deductive analytic approaches, predefined themes, drawn from the interview topic guide and research questions, are used to direct this searching.

Themes and categories must be labelled or 'coded' in a way that facilitates retrieval. Early labels often use the participants' language or terminology and sometimes interesting or unfamiliar terms used by the group studied can form the basis of analytical categories. For example, Becker and Geer's classic study of medical school training uncovered the specialised use of the term 'crock' to denote patients who were seen as less worthwhile to treat by medical staff and students [7].

Labelling needs to be inclusive; categories are added to reflect as many of the nuances in the data as possible, rather than reducing them to a few numerical codes. It is also to be expected that sections of the data – such as discrete incidents – will include multiple themes and are thus coded to several categories. This initial data management is a lengthy and sometimes tedious process, but it allows the researcher to group and link items of data that can then be sorted or arranged under a manageable number of thematic or conceptual headings. It is important to have some system of indexing that records the emerging themes and allows the analysis of data items that fit into more than one category. A number of computer software packages have been developed to facilitate this aspect of the analytical process (see below for the use of software for qualitative analysis).

At this stage, there is likely to be considerable overlap and repetition between the categories. Informed by the analytical and theoretical ideas developed during the research, these categories are further refined and reduced in number by being grouped together. It is then possible to select key themes or categories for further investigation. In the study mentioned earlier, Becker and Geer pursued the use of the term 'crock' by medical students to see what types of patients it described and when and how it was used. This meant collating all the instances when 'crock' occurred in the data. Using these data, Becker and Geer were able to explain how medical students and staff categorised patients according to their utility for teaching/ learning purposes. Once this was established, it became clear why 'crocks' (typically the elderly patient, or the homeless alcoholic) who offered little or no possibility for learning about new or interesting disorders, were treated with disdain.

Grouping categories together typically entails a process of cutting and pasting – selecting sections of data on like or related themes and putting them together. The mechanics of how to do this vary. In the past, multiple copies of notes or transcripts were used so that sections could be, literally, cut out and pasted next to each other or sorted into different piles. Another approach is to write out relevant chunks of data onto index cards that can be grouped in a card filing system. It is also possible to create matrices or spreadsheets to facilitate this process. Whilst considered somewhat old-fashioned, this repeated physical contact and handling of the data has much to recommend it; the process of re-reading the data and sorting it into categories means that the researcher develops an intimate knowledge of the data, even if the process is laborious.

Word processors can be enormously helpful in searching large amounts of text for specific terms. While it is unlikely to be the sole focus of a qualitative research project, the simple frequency with which particular words or phrases appear in a piece of text can be illuminating. Word processing functions can offer considerable advantages to researchers who would have traditionally used annotations in the margins of fieldnotes or interview transcripts, coloured pens, scissors and glue, card systems and paper files. By typing labels directly into the computer file containing the textual data, the 'search' function can be used to gather chunks of text, which can then be copied and pasted. The split screen functions make this a particularly appealing method for sorting and copying data into separate analytic files. For those that do not wish to use computer software, a large table, floor space or white board that can be 'pasted' with notes or cards summarising data can be a helpful way of dealing with the mass of data at this stage.

Once the data are sorted, there are different ways the analysis can proceed. Below, are three broad approaches that are used in health-related research.

Thematic analysis

This can be the simplest form of analysis and, perhaps for this reason, it is the most commonly used in health care research. The researcher groups the data into themes, and examines all the cases in the study to make sure that all the manifestations of each theme have been accounted for and compared. If the purpose of the research is exploratory, or a very small part of a mixed-methods study, these thematic groupings may be simply reported or described at this stage. However, a stronger analysis will move beyond simple description to examine how the themes are interconnected. This involves trying to identify relationships between themes. Sometimes the connections are obvious (e.g. only people from a certain social class or ethnic group hold particular views). At other times, it may be necessary to ask questions of the data to see how the themes are linked; for example, it is often worth looking for gender or age differences in respondents' accounts, or different responses to similar types of events (e.g. a crisis, or critical incident).

In this way thematic analysis can be used to develop taxonomies or classifications, or to develop models or diagrams that express the connections between themes.

Thematic analysis often includes themes that are anticipated (e.g. through reviewing the literature the researcher might be prompted to ask about particular issues) as well as those that emerge (i.e. that arise, directly or indirectly, during the fieldwork). For example, Chapple and Ziebland [8] did not anticipate that humour would play a large part in men's narrative interview accounts of their experiences of testicular cancer. However, it became clear that the use of humour helped men to demonstrate that they were confident that they would recover (testicular cancer is eminently treatable) as well as to affirm that they were still 'one of the lads'. Humour emerged as an important theme in the interviews and led the authors to examine their data in the light of sociological and anthropological literature on the role of humour and explore the various roles that humour had for these men.

Grounded Theory

Glaser and Strauss [9] coined the term *grounded theory* to describe the inductive process of coding incidents in the data and identifying analytical categories as they 'emerge from' the data (developing hypotheses from the 'ground' or research field upwards rather than defining them in advance). The process is very similar to an inductive thematic analysis, but a central feature of grounded theory is that it is cyclical and iterative – the analysis feeds into subsequent sampling, further data collection and the testing of emerging theories. Thus *theoretical sampling* is an important component of grounded theory – this allows the researcher to deliberately select new respondents or settings to test the emerging analytical categories and theories. The analytical process is undertaken until the point of *saturation* when no further analytical constructs can be identified.

In practice, grounded theory is usually a mixture of induction and some deduction, moving between data and theory – which some researchers describe as 'modified grounded theory'. The process of labelling or coding data in the initial phase begins with *open coding* that involves examining the data line by line to identify as many codes as possible. The properties and dimensions of these codes are then examined by asking of each 'what are its characteristics?' and 'what forms does it take?'. *Axial coding* is then used to identify the relationships between codes and *selective coding* to move towards the development of analytical categories by incorporating more abstract and theoretically based elements. A process called *constant comparison* is used to check or compare each coded data item with the rest of the data to establish these analytical categories. In addition, during the coding process, the researcher constructs a series of *memos*, in effect analytical 'notes-to-self', that describe ideas about the data, definitions of codes and their properties, as well as ideas for further sampling and testing. Using these techniques the researcher can slowly build theory or explanations and at the same time test these emerging ideas. Grounded theory can provide rich, detailed interpretations. For example, Glaser and Strauss [10] were able to use this approach to theorise the nature of relationships between patients with terminal illness and their nurses. The type of care given was related to different levels of awareness of dying, which ranged from open awareness (where both patient and nurse openly acknowledge that the patient is dying), through suspicion (on the part of the patient), mutual deception (where both parties pretend that the patient does not know) and closed awareness (where the patient is not aware that she/he is dying).

Unfortunately, the term 'grounded theory' has often been misused as a synonym for any sort of qualitative 'analysis', and sometimes weak analysis at that. It is not uncommon for research papers to report using 'grounded theory', but without any sign of the elements described above. The flexibility required to enable adequate theoretical sampling and continual re-analysis can take a long time. In addition, the fact that it is seldom possible to specify precisely the dimensions or direction of the research at the outset when adhering to a true 'grounded theory' approach can make such projects appear problematic for research funders and ethical committees (see Chapter 6 on ethical issues).

Framework

The *framework approach* developed by the National Centre for Social Research in the United Kingdom is a more deductive form of analysis that is increasingly being used in health care research [11]. It is a development of the matrix-based methods of analysis described by Miles and Huberman [4]. Framework is especially suited to applied or policy research in which the objectives of the investigation are typically set in advance and shaped by the information requirements of the funding body (e.g. a health authority) rather than emerging from a reflexive research process. The timescales of such research may be shorter than other types of research and there tends to be a need to link the qualitative analysis to findings from quantitative investigation. For these reasons, although framework is heavily based in the original accounts and observations of the people studied (i.e. it is 'grounded' and inductive), it starts deductively from the aims and objectives already set for the study. It is systematic and designed for transparency so that the analytic process and interpretations can be viewed and assessed by people other than the primary analyst (see Chapter 8 on quality in qualitative research for more on this issue).

The topic guide used to collect data under the framework approach (e.g. to guide depth interviews) tends to be slightly more structured from the outset than would be the norm for most qualitative research. The analytical process is similar to thematic analysis, but tends to be more explicit and more strongly informed by *a priori* reasoning. Framework analysis has five stages (see Box 7.1). First the researcher *familiarises* him/herself with the data by reading and re-reading the notes and transcripts. He/she then creates a list of the anticipated and emerging themes that can be placed within a *thematic framework* – a series of thematic headings sorted hierarchically into main and sub-themes. These headings are used to label or *index* the original data (some analysts assign numbers to the various headings to facilitate this, others use words or phrases). The initial thematic framework and index terms are likely to be refined as the analysis progresses and it is important to record this developmental work. Once the themes have been identified, they are grouped and sorted, and the original data are distilled into summaries and used to create *charts*. These describe each theme in a matrix format, displaying sub-themes across the columns and each case as a separate row. These charts can be created on

Box 7.1 The five stages of data analysis using the framework approach [11]

- *Familiarisation* – immersion in the raw data (or typically a pragmatic selection from the data) by listening to tapes, reading transcripts, studying notes and so on, to list key ideas and recurrent themes
- *Identifying a thematic framework* – identifying all the key issues, concepts and themes by which the data can be examined and referenced. This is carried out by drawing on *a priori* issues and questions derived from the aims and objectives of the study as well as issues raised by the respondents themselves and views or experiences that recur in the data. The end product of this stage is a detailed index of the data, which labels the data into manageable chunks for subsequent retrieval and exploration
- *Indexing* – applying the thematic framework or index systematically to all the data in textual form by annotating the transcripts with numerical codes from the index, usually supported by short text descriptors to elaborate the index heading. Single passages of text can often encompass a large number of different themes each of which has to be recorded, usually in the margin of the transcript
- *Charting* – rearranging the data according to the appropriate part of the thematic framework to which they relate and forming charts. For example, there is likely to be a chart for each key subject area or theme with entries for several respondents. Unlike simple cut and paste methods that group verbatim text, the charts contain distilled summaries of views and experiences. Thus the charting process involves a considerable amount of abstraction and synthesis
- *Mapping and interpretation* – using the charts to define concepts, map the range and nature of phenomena, create typologies and find associations between themes with a view to providing explanations for the findings. The process of mapping and interpretation is influenced by the original research objectives as well as by the themes that have emerged from the data themselves.

large sheets of paper, or using spreadsheet or data-management software.

Software packages designed to handle qualitative data

The use of specialist CAQDAS (computer assisted qualitative data analysis software) packages has become widespread in the last few years. Researchers now face the decision as to which of several packages they might choose for their study. For up to date information about CAQDAS and courses in the United Kingdom, the independent networking project at the University of Surrey is a useful source, providing a helpful paper, 'Choosing a CAQDAS package', which is on its website at http://caqdas.soc.surrey.ac.uk .

Before making a decision about whether to use CAQDAS and, if so, which software package to buy for a given project, researchers are well advised to visit the software developer's website to explore a downloadable demonstration version. If applicable, it is also a good idea to find out whether other researchers in one's department or locality have experience with similar packages. Considerations might also include whether there will be a team working on the data together, or whether data are all text-based or include images, or audio or video files. Software packages are increasingly able to handle large datasets based on digital audio and video data, which may mean that the preparation of data as written text becomes unnecessary for some studies.

Software packages that have been designed to assist in the analysis of unstructured textual data all have code and retrieval functions. Other functions include the ability to conduct selective retrievals and examine reports separately by any other indexing term (e.g. the respondent's use of a particular term or a shared characteristic such as gender); to use algorithms to identify co-occurring codes in a range of logically overlapping or hierarchically arrayed possibilities; to attach annotations to sections of the text as 'memos'; to add new codes; and to join together existing codes. CAQDAS packages also offer functions that enable far more complex organisation, annotation, data linkage and retrieval of data than was possible with the earliest versions, let alone that which is possible through use of standard word processing packages. Newer versions of software such as Atlas Ti [12], NVivo [13] and HyperResearch [14] also allow for multi-media data files, such as digital video, audio or photographs to be included in the analysis.

It has been suggested that computer-assisted analysis can help the researcher to build theoretical links, search for exceptions and examine 'crucial cases' where counter evidence might be anticipated. A systematic search for disconfirming evidence can be assisted by using Boolean operators (such as 'or', 'and', 'not') to examine the data. An examination of the context of data extracts may be achieved either through considering which other index terms are attached to the data or by displaying the immediate context of the extract by including the lines of text that surround it. This function should particularly appeal to researchers who are concerned about the 'decontextualisation' that can result from fragmenting the data into coded chunks.

Specialist software has been welcomed for its potential to improve the rigour of analysis [15] and certainly can help with some of the more laborious aspects of data retrieval once the data have been coded. There are many potential benefits of using a software package to help with the more laborious side of textual analysis, but some caution is advisable. Some qualitative researchers who have tried CAQDAS packages have disliked the apparent segmentation of the data that can occur, and are concerned that the analysis can lose touch with the context in which the data were generated – although this is not an inevitable by-product of using the packages. It is also important to note that the packages do not provide the researcher with a methodological or analytic framework, and can only assist the analytic process, not design it. While the ability to index, gather and sort are basic and important functions for organising and accessing the data, they are only the initial stages in qualitative analysis.

The prospect of computer-assisted analysis may persuade researchers (or those who fund them) that they can manage much larger amounts of data and increase the apparent 'power' of their study. Qualitative studies, which are not designed to be *numerically* (statistically) representative, may gain little from an expanded sample size except a more cumbersome dataset. The nature and size of the sample should be directed by the research question and analytic requirements, not by the available software. In some circumstances, a single case study design may be the most successful way of generating theory. Lee and Fielding [16] also warn against the assumption that using a computer package will make analysis less time consuming. This may or may not be the case, although it is hoped that it may make the process more demonstrably systematic.

Developing explanations – the role of the researcher

The essential tasks of studying the raw data (e.g. transcripts of interviews), recognising and refining the concepts and coding the data are inescapably the work of the researcher. For these reasons, it is important to dispel the notion that software packages are designed to deliver qualitative analysis of textual and other data. A computer package may be a useful aid when gathering together chunks of data, establishing links between the fragments, organising and reorganising the display and helping to find exceptions, but no package is capable of perceiving a link or defining an appropriate structure for the analysis. To take the analysis beyond the most basic descriptive exercise requires the researcher's analytical skills in moving towards hypotheses or propositions about the data.

The different analytical approaches described provide ways of sorting, arranging and displaying data to assist the search for patterns, linkages and relationships within the data as a way of building explanations. To do this the researcher must ask, 'what lies behind this pattern?' and 'why does this relationship occur?'. The search for deviant cases can be helpful here – it is often the exception or outlier that illuminates the rule or connection binding the other respondents or cases together. For example, in Chapple and Ziebland's study [8] of humour in coping with the experience of testicular cancer, the few men who said that they had felt upset when others used humour were those who had lost both testicles or had been unable to preserve their fertility. This helped the authors to understand the distinction between 'pure' (e.g. jokes about the condition) and 'applied' humour (where jokes served a function – reassuring the man that he was being treated normally by his friends, establishing camaraderie and so on).

Building explanations is a difficult process. It requires intimate knowledge of the data, creativity and lateral thinking. Knowledge of the wider literature – other studies in the area, relevant theories and sometimes apparently unrelated work – plays a central role in this. For example, a key piece one of us used to theorise about hospital waiting lists [17] was a paper about Eastern Bloc bread shop queues [18].

One way of developing explanations is *analytic induction*. Linked to grounded theory this involves an iterative testing and retesting of theoretical ideas using the data. Bloor [19] describes in some detail how he used this procedure to reconstruct the decision-making rules used by ear, nose and throat surgeons (see Box 7.2). In essence, the researcher examines a set of cases, develops hypotheses or constructs and examines further cases to test these propositions – not unlike the statistical tests of association used in quantitative research. In qualitative research, analysis is often carried out by a single researcher. However, some qualitative researchers have given attention to the notion that qualitative analyses may carry greater weight when they can be shown to be consistent between researchers (particularly when the research has been undertaken to inform policy makers) (see Chapter 8). This is close to the concept of inter-rater reliability, which is familiar in quantitative research. For example, Daly *et al.*'s study of cardiac diagnosis [20], and Waitzkin [21] used

---

Box 7.2 Stages in the analysis of fieldnotes in a qualitative study of ear, nose and throat surgeons' disposal decisions for children referred for possible tonsillectomy and adenoidectomy (T&A) [19]

1 Provisional classification – For each surgeon all cases categorised according to the disposal category used (e.g. T&A or tonsillectomy alone)
2 Identification of provisional case features – Common features of cases in each disposal category identified (e.g. most T&A cases were found to have three main clinical signs present)
3 Scrutiny of deviant cases – Include in (2) or modify (1) to accommodate deviant cases (e.g.T&A performed when only two of three signs present)
4 Identification of shared case features – Features common to other disposal categories (e.g. history of several episodes of tonsillitis)
5 Derivation of surgeons' decision rules – From the common case features (e.g. case history more important than physical examination)
6 Derivation of surgeons' search procedures (for each decision rule) – The particular clinical signs looked for by each surgeon
Repeat **2** to **6** for each disposal category

more than one analyst to improve their analyses. However, the appropriateness of the concept of inter-rater reliability in qualitative research is contested. Some qualitative researchers claim that as a qualitative account cannot be held straightforwardly to represent the social world (just as all research findings reflect the identity of the researcher), different researchers are bound to offer different accounts, especially if the data are relatively unstructured. Another, less radical, assertion is that each researcher has unique insights into the data, which cannot be straightforwardly checked by others [22]. For example, the perspectives of colleagues from other disciplinary backgrounds can often add analytic depth to data interpretation and it would seem foolish to ignore such insights simply because they do not concur with the researcher's own.

Armstrong *et al.* [23] attempted to answer the question: do qualitative researchers show consistency in their accounts of the same raw data? To test this, they asked six experienced qualitative researchers independently to analyse a single focus group transcript and to identify and rank in order of salience the major themes emerging in the discussion. Another social scientist, who had not read the transcript of the focus group, then read the six reports to determine the main themes and to judge the extent to which the six researchers agreed. There was quite close agreement about the identity of the basic themes, but the six researchers 'packaged', or linked and contextualised the themes differently. Armstrong *et al.* concluded that such reliability testing was limited by the inherent nature of the process of qualitative data analysis. On the other hand, the interpretations of the six researchers had much in common despite the fact that they were from two different countries (Britain and the United States), and from three different disciplines (anthropology, psychology and sociology). By deliberately selecting a diverse range of analysts (albeit all experienced), Armstrong *et al.* constructed a tough test of inter-rater agreement and one which would be unusual in a typical research study. It would be interesting to see the same exercise repeated with quantitative data, and analysis and analysts from three different social science disciplines!

Despite the potential limitations of the term 'reliability' in the context of qualitative research highlighted by Armstrong *et al.*, there may be merit in involving more than one analyst in situations where researcher bias (i.e. a lack of validity) is especially likely to be perceived to be a risk by others; for example, where social scientists are investigating the work of clinicians or evaluating government policy.

In their study of the contribution of echocardiography to the social process of diagnosing patients with suspected cardiac abnormalities, Daly *et al.* [20] developed a modified form of qualitative analysis involving both the sociologist researchers and the cardiologists who had managed the patients. The raw data consisted of transcripts of the consultations between the patients and the cardiologists, cardiologists' responses to a structured questionnaire and transcripts of open-ended research interviews with the cardiologists and with the patients.

First, the transcripts and questionnaire data were analysed by the researchers to make sense of the process of diagnosis, including the purpose of the test. From this analysis, the researchers identified the main aspects of the consultations that appeared to be related to the use of echocardiography. Next, these aspects or features of the clinical process were turned into criteria in relation to which other analysts could generate their own assessments of the meaning of the raw data. The cardiologists involved then independently assessed each case using the raw data to produce an account of how and why a test was or was not ordered and with what consequences. The assessments of the cardiologists and sociologists were compared statistically (an unusual procedure for a qualitative study) and the level of agreement was shown to be good. Finally, in cases where there was disagreement between the original researchers' analysis and that of the cardiologist, a further researcher repeated the analysis. Remaining discrepancies were resolved by consensus after discussion between the researchers and the cardiologists.

Although there was an element of circularity in part of this lengthy process (in that the formal criteria used by the cardiologists were derived from the initial researchers' analysis) and it involved the derivation of quantitative gradings and statistical analysis of inter-rater agreement, which are unusual in a qualitative study, it meant that clinical critics could not argue that the findings were simply based on the subjective judgements of an individual researcher.

Conclusion

This chapter has shown that analysing qualitative data is not a simple or quick task. Done properly, it is systematic and rigorous, and therefore labour-intensive for the researcher(s) involved and time consuming. Fielding contends that 'good qualitative analysis is able to document its claim to reflect some of the truth of a phenomenon by reference to systematically gathered data'; in contrast, 'poor qualitative analysis is anecdotal, unreflective, descriptive without being focused on a coherent line of inquiry' [24: 168–169]. At its heart, good qualitative analysis relies on the skill, vision and integrity of the researcher doing the analysis, and as Dingwall *et al.* have pointed out, this may require highly trained and, crucially, experienced researchers [25].

Further reading

Emerson RM, Fretz RI & Shaw LL. *Writing Ethnographic Fieldnotes* (Chicago Guides to Writing, Editing, and Publishing) Chicago: University of Chicago Press, 1995.
Ritchie J & Lewis J. *Qualitative Research Practice: A Guide for Social Scientists and Researchers.* SAGE, London, 2003.

References

1. Lapadat JC & Lindsay AC. Transcription in research and practice: from standardisation of technique to interpretive positionings. *Qualitative Inquiry* 1999; **5**: 64–86.
2. Economic and Social Research Council. QUALIDATA: Qualitative Data Archival Resource Centre, established 1994, University of Essex. www.esds.ac.uk/qualidata/about/introduction.asp last accessed 20.03.06.
3. Becker HS. *Sociological Work.* Allen Lane, London, 1971.
4. Miles M & Huberman A. *Qualitative Data Analysis.* SAGE, London, 1984.
5. Silverman D. Going private: ceremonial forms in a private oncology clinic. *Sociology* 1984; **18**: 191–202.
6. Spencer J, Ritchie J & O'Connor W. Analysis: practices, principles and processes. In: Ritchie J & Lewis J, eds. *Qualitative Research Practice: A Guide for Social Scientists and Researchers.* SAGE, London, 2003.
7. Becker HS & Geer B. Participant observation: the analysis of qualitative field data. In: Burgess RG, ed. *Field Research: A Sourcebook and Field Manual.* Allen and Unwin, London, 1982.
8. Chapple A & Ziebland S. The role of humour for men with testicular cancer. *Qualitative Health Research* 2004; **14**: 1123–1139.
9. Glaser BG & Strauss AL. *The Discovery of Grounded Theory.* Aldine, Chicago, IL, 1967.
10. Glaser BG & Strauss AL. *Awareness of Dying.* Aldine, Chicago, IL, 1965.
11. Ritchie J & Lewis J, eds. *Qualitative Research Practice: A Guide for Social Scientists and Researchers.* SAGE, London, 2003.
12. Muhr T. *ATLAS/Ti for Windows*, 1996.

13. Richards T & Richards L. *QSR NUD*IST V3.0*. SAGE, London, 1994.
14. ResearchWare, *Inc. HyperRESEARCH* 2.6. Randolf, MA. 2005. www.researchware.com last accessed 30.12.05.
15. Kelle U, ed. *Computer-Aided Qualitative Data Analysis: Theory, Methods and Practice*. SAGE, London, 1995.
16. Lee R & Fielding N. User's experiences of qualitative data analysis software. In: Kelle U, ed. *Computer Aided Qualitative Data Analysis: Theory, Methods and Practice*. SAGE, London, 1995.
17. Pope C. Trouble in Store: Some thoughts on the management of waiting lists. *Sociology of Health and Illness* 1991; **13**(2): 193–212.
18. Czwartosz Z. On queueing. *Archives Europeenes de sociologie* 1988; **29**: 3–11.
19. Bloor M. On the analysis of observational data: a discussion of the worth and uses of inductive techniques and respondent validation. *Sociology* 1978; **12**: 545–552.
20. Daly J, McDonald I & Willis E. Why don't you ask them? A qualitative research framework for investigating the diagnosis of cardiac normality. In: Daly J, McDonald I & Willis E, eds. *Researching Health Care: Designs, Dilemmas, Disciplines*. Routledge, London, 1992: 189–206.
21. Waitzkin H. *The Politics of Medical Encounters*. Yale University Press, New Haven, 1991.
22. Morse JM. Designing funded qualitative research. In: Denzin NK & Lincoln YS, eds. *Handbook of Qualitative Research*. SAGE, London, 1994: 220–235.
23. Armstrong D, Gosling A, Weinman J *et al*. The place of inter-rater reliability in qualitative research: an empirical study. *Sociology* 1997; **31**: 597–606.
24. Fielding N. Ethnography. In: Fielding N, ed. *Researching Social Life*. SAGE, London, 1993: 155–171.
25. Dingwall R, Murphy E, Watson P *et al*. Catching goldfish: quality in qualitative research. *Journal of Health Services Research and Policy* 1998; **3**: 167–172.

CHAPTER 8

Quality in qualitative health research

Nicholas Mays, Catherine Pope

Introduction

Thus far, this book has outlined the main methods used in qualitative research. As noted in Chapter 1, qualitative methods have long been used in the social sciences, but their use in health research is comparatively recent. In the last decade, qualitative methods have been used increasingly in health services research and health technology assessment, and there has been a corresponding rise in the reporting of qualitative research studies in medical, nursing and related journals [1]. Interest in these methods and their wider exposure in the field of health research have led to necessary scrutiny of qualitative research. Researchers from other traditions are increasingly concerned to understand qualitative methods and, most importantly, to examine the claims researchers make about the findings obtained from these methods. The issue of 'quality' in qualitative research is part of a much larger and contested debate about the nature of the knowledge produced by qualitative research, whether its quality can legitimately be judged and, if so, how.

Qualitative research in health and health services has had to overcome prejudice and a number of misunderstandings. For example, some people believe that qualitative research is 'easy' – a soft option that requires no skills or training. In fact, the opposite is more likely to be the case. The data generated by qualitative studies are cumbersome and difficult to analyse, and their analysis requires a high degree of interpretative skill. Qualitative research also suffers from the 'stigma of the small n' [2] because it tends to deal with a small number of settings or respondents and does not seek to be statistically representative. However, strictly speaking, this feature is irrelevant to the strength of the approach.

Nonetheless, the status of all forms of research depends on assessing the quality of the methods used. In the field of qualitative research, concern about assessing quality has manifested itself in the proliferation of guidelines for doing and judging qualitative work, particularly in the health field [3–6]. Those using and funding research have also played an important role in the development of these guidelines as they become increasingly familiar with qualitative methods, but require some means of assessing their quality and of distinguishing 'good' and 'poor' quality research. To this end, the English NHS Research and Development Programme funded a review of qualitative research methods relevant to health technology assessment [7]. However, while the sponsors of this review may have hoped for a small set of simple quality guidelines to emerge, any thoughtful analysis of the issue is inevitably far more complex. Subsequently, the United Kingdom Cabinet Office commissioned a study to develop a framework to guide assessments of the quality of qualitative evaluation research. This project was a response to the fact that the Government was commissioning and using an increasing number of qualitative policy and programme evaluation studies, but without access to any explicitly agreed standards as to what constituted good quality in qualitative research [8].

In outlining some of the most frequently used qualitative methods and demonstrating their contemporary application in health research, Chapters 2–5 of this book have referred to the strengths and limitations of particular methods. This chapter attempts to bring together some of these quality issues, although it cannot do full justice to the wider epistemological debate about the nature of the knowledge generated by different quantitative and qualitative research methods. It outlines two views of how qualitative methods might be judged. It goes on to argue that qualitative research can be assessed with reference to the same broad criteria of quality as quantitative research, although the meaning attributed to these criteria may not be the same and they may be assessed differently. The chapter concludes with a list of questions that can be used as a guide to assessing the quality of a piece of qualitative research derived from the review by Spencer *et al.* and colleagues [8].

Can we use the same quality criteria?

There has been considerable debate among qualitative researchers over whether qualitative and quantitative methods can and should be assessed according to the same quality criteria. The debate is complex because there is an underlying lack of consensus about precisely what qualitative research is and the variety of approaches included under this heading. Other than the total rejection of any quality criteria on the extreme relativist grounds that social reality does not exist independently of human constructions or accounts of that reality, thereby making assessments of 'quality' impossible and irrelevant (see below) [9], it is possible to identify two broad, opposing positions [10]. First, there are those who have argued that qualitative research represents a distinctive paradigm that generates a different type of knowledge from quantitative research. Therefore, different quality criteria should apply, even though 'quality' can be described and assessed. Second, there are those who have argued that there is no separate philosophy of knowledge underpinning qualitative research and so the same criteria in general terms should be applied to qualitative and quantitative research. Within each position, it is possible to see a range of views. Much of the debate within and between these two positions concerns concepts of 'validity' and to a lesser extent of 'reliability' [8]. Concepts of 'validity' include the more obvious notions of the truth and credibility of findings, but can also include notions of the value or worth of the findings of a piece of qualitative research.

Separate and different: the anti-realist position

Advocates of this position argue that as qualitative research represents a distinct paradigm that generates a distinct form of knowledge, it is inappropriate to apply criteria derived from an alternative paradigm. This means that qualitative research cannot and should not be judged by conventional measures of validity (the test of whether the research is true to some underlying reality), generalisability (the degree to which the specifics of the research can be applied more widely to other settings and populations) and reliability (the extent to which the same findings are produced by repeating the research procedures). For those who adopt this anti-realist position, it would also be inappropriate to use mixed or multiple methods in the same study.

At the core of this position is a rejection of what Lincoln and Guba [11] call 'naïve realism' – a belief that there is a single, unequivocal social reality or truth that is entirely independent of the researcher and of the research process. Instead, they suggest that '"truth" is defined as the best informed . . . and most sophisticated . . . construction on which there is consensus (although there may be several constructions extant which simultaneously meet that criterion) . . . the inquirer and the inquired are interlocked in such a way that the findings of an investigation are the *literal creation* of the inquiry process.' [11].

There are still more extreme relativists who hold that there is no basis even for the consensus referred to by Guba and Lincoln and that all research perspectives are unique and each is equally valid in its own terms. The absence of any external standards would clearly make it impossible for one researcher to judge another's research [9]. Yet, as Murphy *et al.* note, in health services research such an extreme relativist position precludes qualitative research from deriving any unequivocal insights relevant to action and would, therefore, command little support among applied health researchers [7].

Those relativists who maintain that separate criteria are required to evaluate qualitative research have put forward a range of different assessment schemes. In part, this is because the choice and relative importance of different criteria of quality depend on the topic and the purpose of the research. If the key question for qualitative researchers is: 'Why do people do what they do?' then for Popay *et al.* research quality relates to the sampling strategy, adequacy of theory, collection and analysis of data, the extent to which the context has been understood, and whether the knowledge generated incorporates an understanding of the nature of subjective meanings in their social contexts [12]. While there may be some broad similarities between quality standards in quantitative and qualitative research – that is, similar concerns with truth, applicability, consistency and neutrality of research – the fundamental differences in the knowledge each approach generates require that quality is assessed differently in the two traditions [13].

Hammersley has attempted to summarise the different quality criteria and concerns of the relativists (or anti-realists), as follows [10]:

- The degree to which substantive and formal theory is produced and the degree of development of such theory
- The novelty of the claims made from the theory
- The consistency of the theoretical claims with the empirical data collected
- The credibility of the account to those studied and to readers

- The extent to which the description of the culture of the setting provides a basis for competent performance in the culture studied
- The extent to which the findings are transferable to other settings
- The reflexivity of the account – that is, the degree to which the effects of the research strategies on the findings are assessed and the amount of information about the research process that is provided to readers.

These criteria are open to challenge. For example, it is arguable whether all research should be concerned to develop theory. At the same time, many of the criteria listed are not necessarily exclusive to qualitative research (e.g. the extent to which findings are transferable), suggesting that there is a case for assessing both qualitative and quantitative research against the same guiding principles, even if that assessment has to be tailored to the type of research.

Using criteria from quantitative research: subtle realism
Hammersley [14] and Kirk and Miller [15] agree that all research involves subjective perceptions and observations, and that different methods will produce different pictures of the social phenomena being studied. However, unlike the anti-realists, they argue that this does not mean that we cannot believe in the existence of phenomena independent of our claims about them; that is, there is some underlying reality that may be studied. The role of qualitative and quantitative research is thus to attempt to represent that reality rather than to imagine that 'the truth' can be attained. Hammersley calls this *subtle realism*. The logic of this position is that there are ways to assess the different perspectives offered by different research processes against each other and against criteria of quality common to both qualitative and quantitative research. Hammersley identifies the common criteria of validity and relevance (by which he means whether research touches on issues that matter to people) as being fundamental [10]. However, the means of assessment may be modified to take account of the distinctive goals of qualitative and quantitative research. For example, qualitative research frequently does not seek to generalise to a wider population for predictive purposes, but seeks to understand specific behaviour in a naturally occurring context. Similarly, reliability, as conventionally defined, may be of little relevance if unique situations cannot be reconstructed or if the setting studied is undergoing considerable social change [16]. Murphy *et al.*'s comprehensive review [7] supports Hammersley's case [10] for assessing such research according

to its validity, defined as the extent to which the account accurately represented the social phenomena to which it referred, and its relevance, defined in terms of the capacity of the research to help some group of practitioners solve the problems they faced. Each broad criterion will be discussed in turn.

Assuring and assessing the validity of qualitative research

There are no mechanical or 'easy' solutions to limit the likelihood that there will be errors in qualitative research. Furthermore, there is no single way to separate out 'good' from 'bad' qualitative research because it is so diverse. However, there are various ways of improving validity, each of which requires the exercise of judgement on the part of the researcher and, ultimately, the reader of the research.

Triangulation

Triangulation involves the comparison of the results from either two or more different methods of data collection (e.g. interviews and observation) or, more simply, from two or more data sources (e.g. interviews with members of different interest groups). The researcher looks for patterns of convergence to develop or corroborate an overall interpretation. Triangulation is generally accepted as a means of ensuring the comprehensiveness of a set of findings. It is more controversial as a genuine test of the truthfulness or validity of a study. The latter test relies on the assumption that any weakness in one method will be compensated by strengths in another. Occasionally, qualitative methods will reveal inadequacies in quantitative measures or show that quantitative results are at odds with observed behaviour. For example, Stone and Campbell's depth interviews in Nepal (mentioned in Chapter 1) revealed attitudes towards abortion and family planning very different from those recorded in formal fertility surveys [17]. Similarly, Meyer's multi-method approach discussed in Chapter 11 highlights the gap between the findings derived from attitudinal scales and everyday talk about, and practice in relation to, lay participation in care on the ward she studied [18]. However, this use of triangulation is contested. Silverman argues that data from different sources can only be used to identify the context-specific nature of differing accounts and behaviour [19]. He points out that discrepancies between different data sources (such as from doctors and their patients) present a problem of adjudication between rival accounts. Thus, triangulation may be better seen as a way of making a study more comprehensive, or of encouraging a more *reflexive* analysis of the data (see below) than as a pure test of validity.

Respondent validation

Respondent validation, or member checking as it is sometimes called, includes a range of techniques in which the investigator's account is compared with the accounts of those who have been investigated to establish the level of correspondence between the two sets. The reactions to the analyses of those studied are then incorporated into the study findings. Lincoln and Guba [11] regard respondent validation as the strongest available check on the credibility of a research project. However, there are limitations to these techniques as validation tests. For example, the account produced by the researcher is designed for a wide audience and will, inevitably, be different from the account of an individual informant simply because of their different roles in the research process. As a result, it is better to think of respondent validation as part of a process of error reduction, which also generates further original data, which, in turn, require interpretation, rather than as a straightforward check on validity [20].

Clear exposition of methods, of data collection and analysis

As the methods used in all types of social research unavoidably influence the objects of enquiry (and qualitative researchers are particularly aware of this), it is important to provide a clear account of the process of data collection and analysis. This is so that readers can judge the evidence upon which conclusions are drawn, taking account of the way that the evidence was gathered and analysed. For example, in an observational study, it would be particularly pertinent to document the period of time over which observations were made and the depth or quality of the researcher's access to the research setting.

A common failing of qualitative research reports is an inadequate account of the process of data analysis (see Chapter 7). This is compounded by the inductive nature of much qualitative work in which prior conceptualisation is largely inappropriate as the aim is to develop new concepts and categories, and identify their inter-relationships through the process of undertaking the research. As a result, the processes of data collection and analysis are frequently interwoven. Nonetheless, by the end of the study, it should be possible to provide a clear account of how early, simpler systems of classification evolved into more sophisticated coding structures and thence into clearly defined concepts and explanations for the data collected. In some situations, it may be appropriate to assess the inter-rater reliability of coding by asking another researcher to independently code some of the raw data using coding criteria previously agreed upon. Where this is not feasible or appropriate (see Chapter 7 on analysis for more on this), it may be preferable to show that a range of potential explanations has been explored to make sense of the data collected. Finally, it is important to include in the written account sufficient data to allow the reader to judge whether the interpretation offered is adequately supported by the data. This is one of the reasons why qualitative research reports are generally longer than those of quantitative studies as it can be difficult to summarise the data that support a concept or explanation economically.

Reflexivity

Reflexivity means sensitivity to the ways in which the researcher and the research process have shaped the data collected, including the role of prior assumptions and experience, which can influence even the most avowedly inductive enquiries. Researchers can keep a personal research diary alongside the data collection and analysis in which to record their reactions to events occurring during the period of the research. They can and should make their personal and intellectual biases plain at the outset of any research reports to enhance the credibility of their findings. The effects of personal characteristics such as age, gender, social class and professional status (e.g. that of doctor, nurse, physiotherapist, sociologist, etc.) on the data collected and the 'distance' between the researcher and those researched also need to be discussed.

Attention to negative cases

As well as exploring alternative explanations for the data collected, a long-established tactic for reducing error is to search for, and discuss, elements in the data that contradict, or appear to contradict, the emerging explanation of the phenomena under study. *Deviant case analysis* helps refine the analysis until it can explain all or the vast majority of the cases under scrutiny. It is similar to the Popperian quest for evidence that disproves established theories in the natural sciences and can help counteract some of the preconceptions that all researchers bring to their research. In this way, it can contribute to increasing the sophistication and credibility of research reports [21]. Another version of deviant or negative case analysis is to attempt to incorporate seemingly different findings from different studies into a more refined, overarching synthesis (see Chapter 13 on qualitative synthesis).

Fair dealing

The final technique for reducing bias in qualitative research is to ensure that the research design explicitly incorporates a wide range of different perspectives so that the viewpoint of one group is never presented as if it represents the sole truth about any situation. Dingwall [22] coined the term 'fair dealing' to describe this process of attempting to be non-partisan; for him, fair dealing marks the difference between social science and 'muck-raking journalism'. However, this concern to deal even-handedly with all those studied is not shared by all researchers. Indeed, there is a long tradition in sociology, dating from the 1920s Chicago School, of adopting the perspective of the 'underdog' against the dominant views of powerful elites [23]. This position has been severely mauled in recent times. Strong scathingly described it as being more concerned with being 'right on' than with being right [24].

Relevance

Hammersley argued that good quality qualitative research has to be relevant in some way to a public concern, though this does not necessarily mean that the research should slavishly adhere to the immediate concerns or problems defined by policy makers, professionals or managers [10]. Research can be 'relevant' when it either adds to knowledge or increases the confidence with which existing knowledge is regarded.

Another important dimension of relevance is the extent to which findings can be generalised beyond the setting in which they were generated. Quantitative researchers frequently criticise qualitative studies for their lack of representativeness and resultant lack of generalisability. However, it is possible to use forms of probability sampling such as stratified sampling techniques in qualitative research to ensure that the range of settings chosen is representative of the population about which the researcher wishes to generalise. Another tactic is to ensure that the research report has sufficient descriptive detail for the reader to be able to judge whether or not the findings apply in other similar settings.

Finally, it has to be recognised that generalisation from qualitative research does not rely exclusively on notions of statistical logic. The extent to which inferences can be drawn from one setting to another depends as much on the adequacy of the explanatory theory on which they are based as on statistical representativeness [21]. Thus the test is whether categories of cases or settings that are theoretically similar behave in the same way rather than cases or settings that are substantively similar. One way of looking at this is to explore the extent to which the sample of cases studied includes the full range of potentially relevant cases. This is *theoretical sampling* in which an initial sample is drawn to include as many as possible of the factors that might affect variability of behaviour, but is then extended, as required, in the light of early findings and emergent theory explaining that behaviour [2]. Under conceptual or theoretical sampling, statistical 'minority' groups are frequently over-represented to test whether the emerging explanations are equally robust when applied to widely differing populations. The full sample, therefore, attempts to include the full range of settings relevant to the conceptualisation of the subject.

The appropriate role for quality guidelines

The hotly contested debate about whether quality criteria should be applied to qualitative research, together with the differences of view between 'experts' about which criteria are appropriate and how they should be assessed, should warn against unthinking reliance on any one set of guidelines either to use when undertaking such research in the first place, or subsequently to judge the quality of research outputs. Most of the individual criteria proposed are not straightforward to assess. Each requires judgements to be made. A number of practical checklists have been published to help with judging the quality of qualitative work [3–6]. The checklists cover a wide range of aspects of research that may potentially be relevant to the rigour of individual qualitative studies of various types.

The most recent and exhaustive is the framework produced by Spencer and her colleagues on behalf of the UK Cabinet Office which is summarised below [8]. It is an attempt to bring some order to the disparate frameworks in existence. The authors systematically reviewed the research literature on concepts, standards and measures of the quality of qualitative research, including all the existing frameworks (they identified 29 written in English in 2002). The research team also interviewed a wide range of qualitative researchers and users of research to produce a framework for assessing qualitative evaluations of social policies and programmes. The framework is based on the perspective, which we share, that the concerns that lie behind conventional (quantitative) conceptions of quality have relevance for qualitative enquiry, but need to be reformulated and assessed differently.

The framework draws heavily on previous quality assessment criteria and checklists, and attempts to build on the most practicable of the approaches to date. The authors emphasise wisely that it is an aid to informed judgement of quality, not a set of rules to be applied invariantly to all qualitative studies. It is most applicable to accounts of evaluative qualitative research that has been undertaken using the commonest methods; namely, individual interviews, focus groups, observation and documentary analysis. Nevertheless, the principles and many of the questions suggested can be applied to research using a wider range of methods (e.g. conversation or linguistic analysis, archival or historical research, multi-media methods, etc.), and, with suitable modification, to non-evaluative research. Though the framework was primarily designed to assess the outputs of completed research, many of the questions can also be used by researchers at different times during the life of a particular research project to help improve its quality or by those preparing or assessing research proposals.

Spencer and colleagues' framework for assessing the quality of qualitative research evidence

The framework comprises a set of guiding principles, a set of appraisal questions and, for each question, a set of quality indicators.

Guiding principles

There are four principles derived from recurrent themes in the literature and interviews conducted that underpin the framework and help structure the set of appraisal questions. The principles indicate that qualitative evaluation research should be:

- *Contributory* in advancing wider knowledge or understanding about policy, practice or theory (close to the notion of 'relevance' discussed above);
- *Defensible in design* by providing a research strategy that can address the questions posed (i.e. the methods of enquiry should be appropriate to the objectives of the study);
- *Rigorous in conduct* through the systematic and transparent collection, analysis and interpretation of qualitative data (this includes the specific techniques for ensuring validity discussed above); and
- *Credible in claim* through offering well-founded and plausible arguments about the significance of the evidence generated.

Appraisal questions

The guiding principles are used to identify 18 appraisal questions to help assess studies. They cover all the key features and processes involved in qualitative studies: design, sampling, data collection, analysis, reporting, reflexivity and neutrality, ethics, auditability and assessment of findings. When assessing completed studies, it is suggested that the findings are appraised first as this will help in assessing the research process that preceded them.

Quality indicators

For each appraisal question, there is a series of quality indicators that point to the kinds of information needed to judge whether or not the quality feature concerned has been achieved. Though the list is fairly detailed (see Table 8.1), it is not intended to be comprehensive in that other indicators may need to be added for specific studies and, in turn, not all the indicators will be relevant to all studies being assessed. Some knowledge of qualitative research and some expertise in using qualitative methods are desirable in using the framework, particularly to determine the relative weight to give to different indicators in the context of specific studies.

The framework

The full details of the framework and its derivation can be found in Spencer *et al.* [8] and Table 8.1 provides a summary of this.

Table 8.1 Framework for assessing qualitative studies, particularly policy evaluations

Features/processes of the study	Appraisal questions	Quality indicators (possible features of the study for consideration)
Findings	1. How credible are the findings?	Findings are supported by data/study evidence Findings 'make sense'; i.e. have a coherent logic Findings are resonant with other knowledge Corroborating evidence is used to support or refine findings (other data sources or other research evidence)
Findings	2. How has knowledge or understanding been extended by the research?	Literature review summarising previous knowledge and key issues raised by previous research Aims and design related to existing knowledge, but identify new areas for investigation Credible, clear discussion of how findings have contributed to knowledge and might be applied to policy, practice or theory development Findings presented in a way that offers new insights or alternative ways of thinking Limitations of evidence discussed and what remains unknown or unclear
Findings	3. How well does the study address its original aims and purpose?	Clear statement of aims and objectives, including reasons for any changes Findings clearly linked to purposes of the study Summary/conclusions related to aims Discussion of limitations of study in meeting aims
Findings	4. How well is the scope for making wider inferences explained?	Discussion of what can be generalised to the wider population from which the sample was drawn or cases selected Detailed description of the contexts in which the data were collected to allow assessment of applicability to other settings

Findings	Discussion of how propositions/findings may relate to wider theory and consideration of rival explanations
	Evidence supplied to support claims for wider inference
	Discussion of limitations on drawing wider inferences
5. How clear is the basis of evaluative appraisal? *(only relevant to evaluations)*	Discussion of how evaluative judgements (e.g. of effectiveness) have been reached
	Description of any formal appraisal criteria used
	Discussion of nature and source of any divergence in evaluative appraisals
	Discussion of any unintended consequences of policy/intervention, their impact and why they arose
6. How defensible is the research design?	Discussion of how the overall research strategy was designed to meet the aims of the study
	Discussion of rationale for study design
	Convincing argument for specific features/components
	Use of different features and data sources as evidence in findings presented
	Discussion of limitations of design and their implications for evidence produced
7. How well defended is the sample design or target selection of cases/documents?	Description of study locations, and how and why chosen
	Description of population of interest and how sample selection relates to it
	Rationale for selection of target sample, settings or documents
	Discussion of how sample/selections allowed necessary comparisons to be made
8. How well is the eventual sample composition/case inclusion described?	Detailed description of achieved sample/cases covered
	Efforts taken to maximise inclusion of all groups
	Discussion of any missing coverage in achieved samples/cases and implications for study evidence
	Documentation of reasons for non-participation among samples approached or cases selected
	Discussion of access and methods of approach, and how these might have affected coverage

Table 8.1 Continued

Features/processes of the study	Appraisal questions	Quality indicators (possible features of the study for consideration)
Data collection	9. How well were the data collected?	Discussion of who collected the data; procedures and documents used; checks on origin, status and authorship of documents Audio or video recording of interviews, focus groups, discussions, etc. (if not, were justifiable reasons given?) Description of conventions for taking fieldnotes Description of how fieldwork methods may have influenced data collected Demonstration, through portrayal and use of data that depth, detail and richness were achieved in collection
Analysis	10. How well has the analysis been conveyed?	Description of form of original data (e.g. transcripts, observations, notes, documents, etc.) Clear rationale for choice of data management method, tools or package Evidence of how descriptive analytic categories, classes, labels, etc. were generated and used Discussion, with examples, of how any constructed analytic concepts, typologies, etc. were devised and used
Analysis	11. How well are the contexts of data sources retained and portrayed?	Description of background, history and socioeconomic/organisational characteristics of study sites/settings Participants' perspectives/observations are placed in personal context (e.g. use of case studies, vignettes, etc. are annotated with details of contributors) Explanation of origins of written documents Use of data management methods that preserve context (i.e. facilitate within case analysis)
Analysis	12. How well has diversity of perspectives and content been explored?	Discussion of contribution of sample design/case selection to generating diversity Description of diversity/multiple perspectives/alternative positions in the evidence displayed Evidence of attention to negative cases, outliers or exceptions (deviant cases) Typologies/models of variation derived and discussed

Analysis	13. How well has detail, depth and complexity (i.e. richness) of the data been conveyed?	Examination of reasons for opposing or differing positions Identification of patterns of association/linkages with divergent positions/groups Use and exploration of contributors' terms, concepts and meanings Portrayal of subtlety/intricacy within data Discussion of explicit and implicit explanations Detection of underlying factors/influences Identification of patterns of association/conceptual linkages within data Presentation of illuminating textual extracts/observations
Reporting	14. How clear are the links between data, interpretation and conclusions?	Clear conceptual links between analytic commentary and presentation of original data (i.e. commentary relates to data cited) Discussion of how/why a particular interpretation is assigned to specific aspects of data, with illustrative extracts to support this Discussion of how explanations, theories and conclusions were derived; how they relate to interpretations and content of original data; and whether alternative explanations were explored Display of negative cases and how they lie outside main propositions/theory; or how propositions/theory were revised to include them
Reporting	15. How clear and coherent is the reporting?	Demonstrates link to aims/questions of study Provides a narrative or clearly constructed thematic account Has structure and signposting that usefully guide reader Provides accessible information for target audiences Key messages are highlighted or summarised

Table 8.1 Continued

Features/processes of the study	Appraisal questions	Quality indicators (possible features of the study for consideration)
Reflexivity and neutrality	16. How clear are the assumptions, theoretical perspectives and values that have shaped the research and its reporting?	Discussion/evidence of main assumptions, hypotheses and theories on which study was based and how these affected each stage of the study Discussion/evidence of ideological perspectives, values and philosophy of the researchers and how these affected methods and substance of the study Evidence of openness to new/alternative ways of viewing subject, theories or assumptions Discussion of how error or bias may have arisen at each stage of the research, and how this threat was addressed, if at all Reflections on impact of researcher(s) on research process
Ethics	17. What evidence is there of attention to ethical issues?	Evidence of thoughtfulness/sensitivity to research contexts and participants Documentation of how research was presented in study settings and to participants Documentation of consent procedures and information provided to participants Discussion of how anonymity of participants/sources was protected, if appropriate or feasible Discussion of any measure to offer information, advice, support, etc. after the study where participation exposed need for these Discussion of potential harm or difficulty caused by participation and how avoided
Auditability	18. How adequately has the research process been documented?	Discussion of strengths and weaknesses of data sources and methods Documentation of changes made to design and reasons; implications for study coverage Documents and reasons for changes in sample coverage, data collection, analysis, etc. and implications Reproduction of main study documents (e.g. interview guides, data management frameworks, letters of invitation)

Adapted from Spencer *et al.* [8: 22–28] Crown Copyright.

Conclusion

Although the issue of quality in qualitative health and health services research has received considerable attention, as late as 1998, Dingwall and colleagues were able to argue, legitimately, that 'quality in qualitative research is a mystery to many health services researchers' [25]. This chapter has shown how of late qualitative researchers have endeavoured to remedy this deficiency in their research and in devising frameworks for assessing the quality of studies. It has outlined the broad debates about the nature of the knowledge produced by qualitative research and indicated some of the main ways in which the validity and relevance of qualitative studies can be assured. Finally, it has set out the most recent and arguably one of the most comprehensive frameworks for assessing the quality of qualitative studies.

As in quantitative research, the basic strategy to ensure rigour, and thus quality, in qualitative research, is systematic, self-conscious research design, data collection, interpretation and communication. Qualitative research has much to offer. Its methods can, and do, enrich our knowledge of health and health care. It is not, however, an easy option or the route to a quick answer. As Dingwall *et al.* conclude, 'qualitative research requires real skill, a combination of thought and practice and not a little patience' [25].

Further reading

Murphy E, Dingwall R, Greatbatch D, Parker S & Watson P. Qualitative research methods in health technology assessment: a review of the literature. *Health Technology Assessment* 1998; **2**(16).

Spencer L, Ritchie J, Lewis J & Dillon L. *Quality in Qualitative Evaluation: A Framework for Assessing Research Evidence.* London: Government Chief Social Researcher's Office, Prime Minister's Strategy Unit, Cabinet Office, 2003. www.strategy.gov.uk

References

1. Harding G & Gantley M. Qualitative methods: beyond the cookbook. *Family Practice* 1998; **15**: 76–79.
2. Faltermaier T. Why public health research needs qualitative approaches: subjects and methods in change. *European Journal of Public Health* 1997; **7**: 357–363.

3. Boulton M & Fitzpatrick R. Qualitative methods for assessing health care. *Quality in Health Care* 1994; **3**: 107–113.

4. Blaxter M. Criteria for evaluation of qualitative research. *Medical Sociology News* 1996; **22**: 68–71.

5. Secker J, Wimbush E, Watson J *et al.* Qualitative methods in health promotion research: some criteria for quality. *Health Education Journal* 1995; **54**: 74–87.

6. Mays N & Pope C. Rigour in qualitative research. *British Medical Journal* 1995; **311**: 109–112.

7. Murphy E, Dingwall R, Greatbatch D *et al.* Qualitative research methods in health technology assessment: a review of the literature. *Health Technology Assessment* 1998; **2**(16).

8. Spencer L, Ritchie J, Lewis J *et al. Quality in Qualitative Evaluation: A Framework for Assessing Research Evidence.* Government Chief Social Researcher's Office, Prime Minister's Strategy Unit, Cabinet Office, London, 2003. http://www.strategy.gov.uk

9. Smith JK. The problem of criteria for judging interpretive inquiry. *Educational Evaluation and Policy Analysis* 1984; **6**: 379–391.

10. Hammersley M. *Reading Ethnographic Research.* Longman, New York, 1990.

11. Lincoln YS & Guba EG. *Naturalistic Inquiry.* SAGE, Newbury Park, CA, 1985: 84.

12. Popay J, Rogers A & Williams G. Qualitative research and the gingerbread man. *Health Education Journal* 1995; **54**: 389–443.

13. Popay J, Rogers A & Williams G. Rationale and standards for the systematic review of qualitative literature in HSR. *Qualitative Health Research* 1998; **8**: 341–351.

14. Hammersley M. *What's Wrong with Ethnography?* Routledge, London, 1992.

15. Kirk J & Miller M. *Reliability and Validity in Qualitative Research.* Qualitative Research Methods Series No 1. SAGE, London, 1986.

16. Seale C & Silverman D. Ensuring rigour in qualitative research. *European Journal of Public Health* 1997; **7**: 379–384.

17. Stone L & Campbell JG. The use and misuse of surveys in international development: an experiment from Nepal. *Human Organisation* 1986; **43**: 27–37.

18. Meyer JE. Lay participation in care in a hospital setting: an action research study. London: University of London, unpublished PhD thesis, 1995.

19. Silverman D. *Interpreting Qualitative Data: Methods for Analysing Talk, Text and Interaction.* SAGE, London, 1993.

20. Bloor M. Techniques of validation in qualitative research: a critical commentary. In: Miller G & Dingwall R, eds. *Context and Method in Qualitative Research.* SAGE, London, 1997: 37–50.

21. Silverman D. Telling convincing stories: a plea for more cautious positivism in case studies. In: Glassner B & Moreno JD, eds. *The Qualitative-Quantitative Distinction in the Social Sciences.* Kluwer Academic, Dordrecht, 1989: 57–77.
22. Dingwall R. Don't mind him — he's from Barcelona: qualitative methods in health studies. In: Daly J, McDonald I & Willis E, eds. *Researching Health Care.* Tavistock/Routledge, London, 1992: 161–75.
23. Guba EG & Lincoln YS. *Fourth Generation Evaluation.* SAGE, Newbury Park, CA, 1989.
24. Strong P. Qualitative sociology in the UK. *Qualitative Sociology* 1988; **11**: 13–28.
25. Dingwall R, Murphy E, Watson P *et al.* Catching goldfish: quality in qualitative research. *Journal of Health Services Research and Policy* 1998; **3**: 167–172.

CHAPTER 9

Combining qualitative and quantitative methods

Alicia O'Cathain, Kate Thomas

Research in health and health care can be solely qualitative or quantitative, or can use a mixed methods approach that involves 'integrating quantitative and qualitative data collection and analysis in a single study or a program of inquiry' [1: 7]. Chapters 10–12 explore some styles of research that do this. A common reason for mixing methods is to expand the scope of enquiry by accessing a wider range of data. Examples include an ethnographic study undertaken alongside a randomised controlled trial of the use of leaflets for promoting informed choice in maternity care to gain a better understanding of how the intervention was delivered in practice [2,3], or in-depth interviews undertaken following a survey of primary care use to explain the patterns of use shown in the survey [4]. Unfortunately, researchers sometimes use the terms 'mixed methods', 'multi-methods' and 'multiple methods' interchangeably. They may mean the use of various combinations of *qualitative* methods within a single study, or the combined use of different *quantitative* methods, or they may mean borrowing a sampling or analysis technique associated with one methodology for use in another. In this chapter, the term 'mixed methods' is used to mean combining qualitative and quantitative components within a single study.

Mixed methods: necessity or impossibility?

To enhance the relevance of policy-related research, policy makers and researchers are broadening the scope of research questions asked. For example, they are no longer willing to address only the specific question of whether interventions work, but also wish to understand how they work, and how best to develop both interventions and evaluations that can be implemented in health care settings. Different methods have different strengths and weaknesses for addressing these questions, with qualitative methods suited to addressing how interventions operate and quantitative methods more suited to assessing whether these interventions are effective. This increasing recognition of the complexity of factors affecting health and health care [5], and the desire to answer a wider range of questions about them, have often made a mixed methods approach a necessity. However, this approach is only appropriate for addressing some sets of research questions, and researchers need to provide an explicit justification as to why a mixed methods approach is appropriate for their study. Designing mixed methods studies just because everyone else seems to be doing so, or funding bodies like them [6], may simply result in 'mixed-up methods'.

While the key justification for using mixed methods in health and health care research is a practical one, some researchers take the stance that methods associated with different theoretical positions or paradigms cannot and should not be mixed. Typically quantitative methods are associated with positivism and ideas about an objective social reality external to the researcher, and qualitative methods with interpretivism and ideas about social reality being constituted through the subjective meanings people attach to phenomena (see Chapter 1). Researchers engaging in mixed methods studies may sidestep such philosophical debates and adopt a pragmatic approach of 'if it works then do it'. Or they may draw on 'subtle realism' (discussed in Chapter 8) which accommodates both qualitative and quantitative methods. Finally they may use the theoretical and methodological differences within a study to generate more insights than would be possible with either method alone [7]. Researchers adopting a pragmatic stance may fail to recognise theoretical and methodological differences until problems arise within a team, for example, if the resulting 'mix' begins to reveal the researchers' different perspectives [8]. It is worth being aware of these differences in perspective within any mixed methods research team from the outset as they underpin different views about data collection, analysis and what constitutes good quality research. It is likely to be important to explore likely differences within the team before embarking on the research.

Ways of combining qualitative and quantitative methods

This chapter aims to show that the careful and purposeful mixing of methods can result in successful research outcomes. Researchers

Box 9.1 Ways of combining qualitative and quantitative methods [9]

Findings from different methods are checked against each other

Qualitative research facilitates quantitative research by generating hypotheses for testing or generating items for a questionnaire

Quantitative research facilitates qualitative research by identifying people to participate in the qualitative enquiry

Qualitative and quantitative research are used together to provide a bigger or richer picture

Quantitative research accesses structural issues whereas qualitative research accesses processes

Quantitative research emphasises the researchers' concerns whereas qualitative research emphasises the subjects' concerns

Quantitative research helps to generalise qualitative findings

Qualitative research facilitates interpretation of findings from quantitative research

have described a variety of ways of combining qualitative and quantitative methods in both health [6] and social research (see Box 9.1) [9]. Mixed method approaches have been used in evaluative and exploratory research, and to develop research instruments.

Mixed methods in the evaluation of health care

Historically, the approach to evaluation in health care in the United Kingdom has been outcomes-focused, using randomised controlled trials, or quasi-experimental designs such as before-and-after studies, to test the effectiveness of interventions. However, there are many examples of mixed methods evaluative studies in health in the United Kingdom [10] and many insightful reflections on this approach in evaluative educational research in the United States [11]. Four approaches to combining methods in a single evaluation study are developing. First, qualitative methods can be used within a process evaluation undertaken alongside a randomised controlled trial (RCT) or other experimental design, using observation and interviews to study how an intervention works in practice.

There are numerous examples of this approach [2,3] and, as importantly, there is a growing literature focusing on the issues arising from researchers' experiences of these studies [12–14]. Second, mainly qualitative action-research methods can be used in a 'formative' evaluation that takes place either prior to, or alongside, a mainly 'summative' evaluation [15]. Here, qualitative research is used to help service providers to develop the intervention *in situ* ('formative' evaluation) while the quantitative research is used to measure whether the intervention has worked ('summative' evaluation). Third, qualitative research can be used to improve the design and conduct of the trial itself, rather than the intervention. In a ground-breaking example, observation and interviews with health professionals recruiting patients for a pilot RCT were used to identify potential barriers to participation in the ensuing trial, and resulted in substantially increased participation rates [16]. Finally, qualitative research can be employed throughout the different phases of the development and evaluation of complex interventions to develop a better understanding of how the interventions might work and improve how they are delivered in practice during the early phases of research [5].

Exploratory research combining survey and qualitative methods

There is a long history of using surveys with a range of qualitative methods in social research [17]. An example from health care is a study of the relationship between need, demand and use of primary care services where Rogers and colleagues used a survey and health diary of 423 people followed by in-depth interviews with 55 survey respondents [4]. The survey and diary analysis produced a sampling frame for the qualitative component. Logistic regression identified people who should have been frequent users because of their health needs but who were not, and those who should not have been frequent users but who were. Rather than survey one group of patients and interview a separate group concurrently, the researchers employed a sequential approach, using the quantitative analysis to identify a sample of such unusual cases for interview that optimised the ability of the qualitative component to generate insights relevant to the research questions. The researchers also drew together the survey and interview responses for the interviewees, analysing the quantitative and qualitative data together as well as separately. The authors concluded that the mixed methods approach had given them a broader understanding of the dynamics of health care use, with the survey showing the extent to which people used self-care in relation to primary care services, while the qualitative component illuminated the ways in which past experience and domestic context affected decision-making. Working between survey and interview data in this way requires particular skills. Mason offers a helpful exploration of the process of making links between survey data and interviews, the techniques for facilitating this process, and the epistemological considerations involved [18].

Using mixed methods in the development of research instruments

Qualitative interviews or focus groups can be used to generate items and language for a questionnaire that will then be used in a survey. The qualitative component of the study is considered to be a mark of quality, ensuring that the questionnaire is both relevant and comprehensible to potential respondents. This relationship has been extended to include cognitive testing in questionnaire design [19] where qualitative interviews are used to assess the validity of questions prior to finalising the questionnaire. A related application is in the development of outcome measures such as indices of health-related quality of life or patient satisfaction. Traditionally, qualitative research has been used only to generate items for inclusion in a new measure. However, more extensive use can be made of the qualitative component to identify underlying concepts that shape both the instrument and its subsequent quantitative psychometric testing [20]. Qualitative research can be used to improve established instruments as well as develop new ones [21]. Additionally, established measurement tools can themselves be used to structure qualitative interviews as a mechanism for gaining a deeper understanding of the meaning of health to particular patient groups [22].

Designing and analysing mixed methods studies

When designing mixed methods studies, researchers need to consider the purpose of mixing methods [11], the priority and sequence of mixing [23], and how and when integration will occur. The purpose of mixing methods may be to address two linked, and equally important, questions. For example 'do leaflets promote informed choice in maternity care and how do they do this (or not) in practice?' [2,3]. Here the methods are used with the intention of *complementarity*, allowing researchers to uncover different perspectives and hence more of the picture. A different purpose is that of *development*, where one method is used explicitly to aid the other – for example, focus groups facilitating the design of a survey questionnaire. Another commonly cited reason for mixing methods is *triangulation* where the findings from two different methods are compared and agreement is sought (see the previous Chapter for more on this). This is problematic as a means of ensuring validity: researchers need to be clear about why different methods with different strengths and weaknesses might be expected to give the same answer, and decide which they will privilege as 'correct' if the answers differ. However, mixed methods approaches may be used as a means of comparing data sets or findings to explore convergence, divergence and contradiction – a process that has also been called *crystallisation* [24]. Here, no *a priori* assumption of convergence is made and apparent contradictions between findings are viewed as 'inter-method discrepancies' that may lead to further valuable insights [17].

The priority and sequence of methods can be used to distinguish different mixed methods designs [23]. Priority denotes whether one method is dominant; for example, the status of a survey may be to generate a sample for a predominantly qualitative study, or both survey and interview study may have equal status. The priority accorded to a component will have implications for resource use, depth of analysis and the dissemination of findings from different components of the study. Methods can be undertaken concurrently, or sequentially. Or there may be an iterative process whereby a qualitative component is used to develop a hypothesis, which is then tested in a survey, which is then followed by a further qualitative component to explore unusual or interesting findings from the survey.

Finally, researchers need to consider when and how links will be made between components within a study. Sometimes this is built into the design; for example, a survey may identify a sample for in-depth interview. Here the link is that the analysis of one method produces a sampling frame for the other method that would otherwise be unavailable or difficult to obtain. Where methods are undertaken concurrently, how and where integration or links between methods will occur will need to be made explicit. According to the definition of mixed methods used here, both data sets will be analysed separately. However, decisions will need to be made about when findings from the two components are to be linked. Crystallisation of findings from both components may be reported in the results or discussion section of a report. Alternatively, integration can happen earlier where the findings of one method affect how the other method is analysed; for example the qualitative component may identify a typology of service provision that can then be used within the quantitative analysis. There is also scope for the raw data from the qualitative and quantitative components to be brought together. For example, the questionnaire and interview transcript for an individual can be compared and patterns looked for across cases. This may involve 'quantifying' qualitative data, that is assigning codes to the presence and absence of themes within individual cases, or turning quantitative data into text for qualitative analysis [8].

Getting the most out of mixed methods studies

Barbour has suggested that mixed methods studies can produce a whole greater than the sum of the parts [6]. Researchers engaged in mixed methods studies may wish to consider what the extra 'yield' has been over and above a qualitative study and a quantitative study undertaken independently. Is the yield a better quantitative instrument, access to a hard-to-reach sample, more or deeper insights, a more focused analysis of one component, a more rounded picture, or more or less confidence in the findings? Researchers sometimes reflect on these issues in the discussion sections of reports, but then publish the qualitative and quantitative components separately. Although there may be practical barriers, researchers need to consider writing mixed methods publications [25], or at least being explicit about the links between methods in publications that focus on results from only one methodological component [26].

Mixing methods in secondary research

This chapter has focused on using mixed methods for primary research. More recently, work has been undertaken exploring the different ways of synthesising evidence from existing qualitative and quantitative studies (see Chapter 13). Researchers can also use a mixture of secondary and primary research – for example, combining a quantitative systematic review (secondary research) with qualitative interviews designed to obtain stakeholders' view of the issue under study (primary research).

Conclusions

Combining qualitative and quantitative methods is an important approach to consider as part of an array of study designs available to researchers. Such mixed methods studies are likely to generate 'added value', but will be challenging as well as rewarding. Researchers may need to engage with the methodological differences that exist within multidisciplinary research teams and work hard to make such studies yield their potential. Successful studies require researchers to be explicit about their rationale for using mixed methods and to take the process of *integration* between methods as seriously as the individual components.

Further reading

Brannen J. ed. *Mixing Methods: Qualitative and Quantitative Research.* Aldershot, Ashgate, 1992.

Creswell JW. *Research Design. Qualitative, Quantitative, and Mixed Methods Approaches,* 2nd edn. SAGE, London, 2003.

Tashakkori A & Teddlie C, eds. *Handbook of Mixed Methods in Social and Behavioural Research.* SAGE, London, 2003.

References

1. Creswell JW, Fetters MD & Ivankova NV. Designing a mixed methods study in primary care. *Annals of Family Medicine* 2004; **2**: 7–12.
2. Stapleton H, Kirkham M & Thomas G. Qualitative study of evidence based leaflets in maternity care. *British Medical Journal* 2002; **324**: 639–643.
3. O'Cathain A, Walters SJ, Nicholl JP *et al.* Use of evidence based leaflets to promote informed choice in maternity care: randomised controlled trial in everyday practice. *British Medical Journal* 2002; **324**: 643–646.
4. Rogers A & Nicolaas G. Understanding the patterns and processes of primary care use: a combined quantitative and qualitative approach. *Sociological Research Online* 1998; **3**: 5.
5. Medical Research Council. *A Framework for Development and Evaluation of RCTs for Complex Interventions to Improve Health.* Medical Research Council, London, 2000.

6. Barbour RS. The case for combining qualitative and quantitative approaches in health services research. *Journal of Health Services Research and Policy* 1999; **4**: 39–43.
7. Greene JC & Caracelli VJ. Defining and describing the paradigm issue in mixed-method evaluation. In: Greene JC & Caracelli VJ, eds. *Advances in Mixed-Method Evaluation: The Challenges and Benefits of Integrating Diverse Paradigms.* Jossey-Bass Publishers, San Francisco, 1997: 5–17.
8. Sandelowski M. Combining qualitative and quantitative sampling, data collection, and analysis techniques in mixed-method studies. *Research in Nursing & Health* 2000; **23**: 246–255.
9. Bryman A. Quantitative and qualitative research: further reflections on their integration. In: Brannen J, ed. *Mixing Methods: Qualitative and Quantitative Research.* Ashgate, Aldershot, 1992: 57–78.
10. Murphy E, Dingwall R, Greatbatch D *et al*. Qualitative research methods in health technology assessment: a review of the literature. *Health Technology Assessment,* 1998; **2**(16): 215–237.
11. Greene JC, Caracelli VJ & Graham WF. Toward a conceptual framework for mixed-method evaluation designs. *Educational Evaluation and Policy Analysis* 1989; **11**: 255–274.
12. Parry-Langdon N, Bloor M, Audrey S *et al*. Process evaluation of health promotion interventions. *Policy & Politics* 2003; **31**: 207–216.
13. Rousseau N, McColl E, Eccles M *et al*. Qualitative methods in implementation research. In: Thorsen T & Markela M, eds. *Changing Professional Practice: Theory and Practice of Clinical Guidelines Implementation.* DSI, Copenhagen, 1999: 99–116.
14. Riley T, Hawe P & Shiell A. Contested ground: how should qualitative evidence inform the conduct of a community intervention trial? *Journal of Health Services Research and Policy* 2005; **10**: 103–110.
15. Bate P & Robert G. Studying health care 'quality' qualitatively: the dilemmas and tensions between different forms of evaluation research within the UK National Health Service. *Qualitative Health Research* 2002; **12**: 966–981.
16. Donovan J, Mills N, Smith M *et al*. Improving design and conduct of randomised trials by embedding them in qualitative research: ProtecT (prostate testing for cancer and treatment) study. *British Medical Journal* 2002; **325**: 766–770.
17. Fielding NG & Fielding JL. *Linking Data.* SAGE, London, 1986.
18. Mason J. Linking qualitative and quantitative data analysis. In: Bryman A & Burgess RG, eds. *Analysing Qualitative Data,* 1994: 89–110.
19. Collins D. Pretesting survey instruments: an overview of cognitive methods. *Quality of Life Research* 2003; **12**: 229–238.
20. Baker R, Preston C, Cheater F *et al*. Measuring patients' attitudes to care across the primary/secondary interface: the development of the patient career diary. *Quality in Health Care* 1999; **8**: 154–160.

21. Paterson C & Britten N. In pursuit of patient-centred outcomes: a qualitative evaluation of the 'Measure Yourself Medical Outcome Profile'. *Journal of Health Services Research and Policy* 2000; **5**: 27–36.
22. Adamson J, Gooberman-Hill R, Woolhead G *et al.* 'Questerviews': using questionnaires in qualitative interviews as a method of integrating qualitative and quantitative health services research. *Journal of Health Services Research and Policy* 2004; **9**: 139–145.
23. Morgan DL. Practical strategies for combining qualitative and quantitative methods: applications to health research. *Qualitative Health Research* 1998; **8**: 362–376.
24. Sandelowski M. Triangles and crystals: on the geometry of qualitative research. *Research in Nursing & Health* 1995; **18**: 569–574.
25. O'Cathain A, Nicholl J, Sampson F *et al.* Do different types of nurses give different triage decisions in NHS Direct? A mixed methods study. *Journal of Health Services Research and Policy* 2004; **9**: 226–233.
26. Donovan JL, Peters TJ, Noble S *et al.* Who can best recruit to randomised trials? Randomised trial comparing surgeons and nurses recruiting patients to a trial of treatments for localized prostate cancer (the ProtecT study). *Journal of Clinical Epidemiology* 2003; **56**: 605–609.

CHAPTER 10

Case studies

Justin Keen

Introduction

The medical approach to understanding disease has traditionally drawn heavily on qualitative data and, in particular, on case studies to illustrate important or interesting phenomena. This chapter discusses the use of qualitative research methods, not in individual clinical care, but in case studies of health service change initiatives. It is useful to understand the principles guiding the design and conduct of these studies, because they are used by organisational inspectorates, such as the Healthcare Commission in England, and to investigate the quality of work of individual doctors and other health professionals. Case studies are also routinely used by the National Audit Office (NAO) [1] in the United Kingdom, and audit offices and regulatory bodies in other countries [2]. Case studies have also been used by researchers in evaluations, such as those of Health Action Zones in the United Kingdom [3], business process re-engineering [4] in hospitals, intermediate care [5], and the processes involved in admitting people to intensive care [6]. Case studies may use a range of qualitative methods including interviews, analysis of documents and non-participant observation of meetings, or they may combine qualitative and quantitative methods (see Chapter 9 for a fuller discussion of combining qualitative and quantitative methods).

This chapter will briefly outline the circumstances where case study research can usefully be undertaken in health service settings. Then, the ways in which qualitative methods are used within case studies are discussed. Illustrative examples are used to show how qualitative methods are applied.

Case study research

Health professionals often find themselves asking important practical questions such as: should we be involved in the management of our local services; and how can we integrate new clinical practices into our work? There are, broadly, two ways in which such questions can usefully be addressed. One is to analyse the proposed policies themselves, by investigating whether they are internally consistent, and by using theoretical frameworks derived from previous research to predict their effects on the ground. For example, it is possible to use this sort of approach to policy analysis to assess the respective merits of the Kaiser Permanente health care system (an integrated health care organisation providing a non-profit health plan across several states in the United States), and the UK NHS [7,8].

The other approach, and the focus of this chapter, is to study policy implementation empirically. Empirical evaluative studies are concerned with placing a value on an intervention or policy change. The empirical evidence is used to help teams to form judgements about the appropriateness of an intervention, and whether the outputs and outcomes of the intervention are justified by their inputs and processes. Asking participants about their experiences, and observing them in meetings and other work settings, can provide rich data for descriptive and explanatory accounts of the ways in which policies and more specific interventions work and their subsequent impact.

Case studies are most valuable where a planned change is occurring in a messy real world setting, and when it is important to understand why such interventions succeed or fail. Many interventions will typically depend for their success on the involvement of several different interested parties, so it is usually necessary to be sensitive to issues of collaboration and conflict, which traditional health services research approaches are not designed to address. The ways in which such policies are normally formulated and promulgated mean that researchers have no control over events. As a result, experimental designs are typically not feasible, and even opportunities for rigorous comparison using observational designs can be limited. Indeed, it is often not clear at the outset whether an intervention will be fully implemented by the end of a study period. One has only to think of accounts of the problems faced in implementing computer systems in health care to appreciate this possibility [9].

Another common problem is that an intervention may be ill-defined, at least at the outset, and so cannot easily be distinguished from the general environment. For example, at the time of writing there is considerable uncertainty about policy innovations such as the nature of general practice-based commissioning in the NHS in England, or the complex structural changes taking place in the financing and delivery of US health care. Indeed, case studies are often concerned with understanding the nature of the intervention as much as with establishing its costs and effects. This helps to explain why case studies tend to be conducted in phases, as research teams have to spend time establishing the nature of an intervention before they can, with confidence, identify the most appropriate empirical tests of the effects of that intervention.

Even where it is well defined, an intervention may not have costs and effects that are easily captured. For example, the networking and other elements of the NHS information technology strategy, 'Connecting for Health', are well defined [10]. However, because the systems will be used by many thousands of people every day, their effects will be felt in many different places and by different groups of people, and thus will be hard to measure. For example, the benefits experienced by people working in hospitals are likely to be different to those experienced by primary care staff. Added to this, our understanding of the ways in which electronic networks influence people's working practices in organisations is poor, and so it is necessary to investigate the causal mechanisms involved, before going on to attempt to attribute any observed effects to the networks. Isolating causal mechanisms is often best achieved using a combination of qualitative and quantitative methods within a case study design.

The design of case studies

Case studies can be undertaken in different ways, but have a number of common features. They start with the identification of research questions that stem from concerns about the implications of new policies, or sometimes from claims about new management theories. Case studies are usually undertaken prospectively, examining the implementation of policies over a period of time. Just as in experimental studies, research teams have to identify research questions, and decide what a good solution would look like if found, so that empirical tests can be identified. Many case studies start by asking broad questions such as: 'What are the intended effects?', and 'What are the important features and relationships that will affect the outcome of this initiative?' In a study of intermediate care in England [5], for example, the research team drew on published findings about earlier policies with similar characteristics, and on policy documents that contained statements about the Government's objectives for intermediate care. The team decided that intermediate care would succeed or fail, in large part, depending on whether or not it led to better integration of services. One of the key questions, therefore, was, 'Does intermediate care promote better integration of services?'. This in turn suggested the broad thrust of the research strategy: the team would need to identify measures of service integration and criteria for deciding whether or not a particular group of services was integrated.

The early fieldwork is designed to generate data that can be used to identify and refine specific research questions inductively. In some ways, the process is similar to the conduct of clinical consultations, in that it involves initial exploration and progress towards a diagnosis inferred from the available data. The evaluation of intermediate care mentioned above provides an example of this approach. The researchers conducted interviews with relevant staff, observed meetings, analysed documents and collected quantitative data on patterns of service use. Over time, the data were used to develop a conceptual framework that captured the essential features of intermediate care, and the framework was then used to identify further research methods that were used to address more precisely posed research questions, and to describe and explain the progress that the study sites had made.

Site selection is important in the case study approach. There are two principal approaches: purposive sampling in which sites are selected on the basis that they are typical of the phenomenon being investigated; and theoretical sampling that is designed specifically to confirm or refute a hypothesis derived either from previous research or data collected earlier in the same study (see Chapter 7, section on 'grounded theory' for more on theoretical sampling) [11]. Qualitative sampling in general is distinct from statistical sampling: the former is concerned with the selection of sites to address a research question, whereas the latter is concerned with identifying a sample that is statistically representative of a population. Researchers can benefit from expert advice from doctors and others with knowledge of the subject being investigated, and can usefully build the possibility of testing findings at further sites into the initial research design. Replication of results across further sites helps to ensure that early findings are not due to idiosyncratic features of the first set of sites selected.

Case studies are typically constructed to allow comparisons to be drawn [12]. The comparison may be between different approaches to implementation of the same policy, or between sites where an innovation is taking place and ones where normal practice prevails. In a recent study of clinical governance [13], the study team investigated differences in the ways in which governance was interpreted and developed in two contrasting services, for coronary heart disease and mental health. The team also selected sites on a purposive basis, to ensure that for each service there were sites that were approaching development in different ways, offering further opportunities for comparison and contrast.

It is never possible to study every aspect of activity at a site from every angle, and choices have to be made about the phenomena within the sites that are most likely to yield answers to the main research questions [14]. In the evaluation of intermediate care, for example, each study site was defined geographically and organisationally, because intermediate care involves a range of services that cover particular geographical patches. Within each site, the case studies focussed on the activities that went into integrating service delivery, and working towards more person-centred care. The evaluation team chose not to look in any detail at the ways in which human resources issues were handled, or at the ways in which finance managers dealt with budgeting issues. These and other issues might well have been interesting in their own right, but investigation of them would not have helped to answer the research questions at hand.

The next step is to select methods. A distinctive feature of case study research is the use of multiple methods and sources of evidence with the aim of ensuring the comprehensiveness of findings as well as potentially strengthening their validity [12]. The use of particular methods is discussed in other chapters of this book. Case studies often use triangulation [15] (see Chapter 8) to attempt to maximise confidence in the validity of findings. It is argued by some that any one method of data collection must produce less valid results than a combination. Using different methods and sources may help to address this problem. However, reservations have been expressed about the use of triangulation in qualitative research as a straightforward technique for improving study validity [16], (see Chapters 8 and 9 for more on this) given that different methods and sources of data will tend to provide different sorts of insights rather than contribute to a single, accumulating picture. It is probably best to regard triangulation between different sources and methods within case studies as a way of making them more comprehensive and encouraging a more reflexive analysis of the data as the analyst can expect to find elements of convergence, divergence and contradiction in the data drawn from different sources and methods.

Some studies have adopted a different approach to validity, and used comparison of case study data with data from a larger sample to explore how far findings might be strengthened and generalised. The evaluation of clinical governance employed this strategy, using survey as well as case study data [12]. Methodological development is still needed in this area to identify robust strategies for combining results from different methods and sites.

An example of the use of multiple methods is provided by a study of the impact of business process re-engineering (BPR) in a teaching hospital in England [4]. Re-engineering is a management theory concerning the way in which organisations should be designed, and stresses the importance of challenging existing working practices that, its advocates argue, are often inefficient and lead to poor quality products or services. Re-engineering involves a fundamental review, and then re-design, of working practices. The researchers decided, on the basis of early fieldwork, that re-engineering needed to be studied in three different contexts in the hospital, namely at the levels of senior management, clinical directorates and clinical service delivery. They further focused on six clinical services where the local implementation team was targeting its efforts, and consciously chose to study different specialties (e.g. at least one elective and one emergency service, and at least one in-patient and one out-patient service). They monitored development over a three-year period, using a range of methods including interviews, review of documents relevant to BPR, and non-participant observation of meetings. The data obtained using each method were analysed separately and then the results compared with one another. By using the same methods in different services and management contexts, the researchers were able to compare and contrast experiences in those settings. Where similar observations were made in a number of different settings, this helped to increase confidence in their findings, partly by helping to account for any idiosyncrasies in particular services.

Data collection should be directed towards the development of an analytical framework that will facilitate the interpretation of findings. Analytical frameworks are, in effect, syntheses of the available evidence, combined in a way that helps to describe and explain how the different elements of the cases being studied fit together. The framework must not be imposed on the data, but derived from them in an iterative process over the course of an evaluation. As the earlier discussion has suggested, the framework should reflect both an understanding of the nature of the intervention and of the ways in which it does – or should – generate changes in costs and benefits. In the evaluation of intermediate care, there was no obvious pre-existing theory that could be drawn upon: the development of an analytical framework during the study was crucial to help organise the data and evaluate findings. The first part of the framework focused on the extent to which intermediate care services were co-ordinated with one another, and provided a simple model in which different services were viewed as being joined together in a network. The empirical evidence showed that all the sites were moving towards more integrated service delivery. The second part of the framework focused on the experiences of the older people who used intermediate care services and the ways in which the services influenced people's well-being.

The investigator is left, finally, with the difficult task of making a judgement about the findings of a study and determining its wider implications. The purpose of the steps followed in designing and building the case study is to maximise confidence in the findings, but interpretation inevitably involves value judgements and the danger of bias. The extent to which research findings can be assembled into a single coherent account of events varies; individual cases may exhibit common characteristics or fare very differently. In some circumstances widely differing opinions of participants are themselves very important, and should be reflected in any report. The case study approach enables the researcher to gauge confidence in both the internal and external validity of the findings, and make comments with the appropriate assurance or with reservations.

Conclusion

The complexity of the issues that health professionals have to address and increasing recognition by policy makers, academics and practitioners of the value of case studies in evaluating health service interventions, suggest that the use of such studies is likely to increase in the future. Their most important use may be by regulators, including bodies in the NHS such as the Healthcare Commission which has made case studies part of the machinery through which doctors and other clinicians are held to account for their work. In policy research, qualitative case study designs can be used to evaluate many policy, management and practice changes that impinge on the lives of clinicians, particularly where those questions are concerned with how or why initiatives take a particular course.

Further reading

Ragin C. *Fuzzy Set Social Science*. University of Chicago Press, Chicago, 2000.

References

1. National Audit Office. *Cost over-runs, funding problems and delays on Guy's Hospital phase III development*. HC 761, Session 1997–98. Stationery Office, London, 1998.
2. Pollitt C, Girre X, Lonsdale J *et al*. *Performance or Compliance? Performance Audit and Public Management in Five Countries*. Oxford University Press, Oxford, 1999.
3. Bauld L, Judge K, Barnes M *et al*. Promoting social change: the experience of Health Action Zones in England. *Journal of Social Policy* 2005; **34**: 427–445.
4. McNulty T & Ferlie E. *Re-Engineering Health Care*. Oxford University Press, Oxford, 2003.
5. Moore J, West R & Keen J. Networks and Governance: The Case of Intermediate Care. Submitted to *Social Policy and Administration*.
6. Martin D, Singer P & Bernstein M. Access to intensive care unit beds for neurosurgery patients: a qualitative case study. *Journal of Neurology, Neurosurgery and Psychiatry* 2003; **74**: 1299–1303.
7. Feachem R, Sekhri N & White L. Getting more for their dollar: a comparison of the NHS with California's Kaiser Permanente. *British Medical Journal* 2002; **324**: 135–141.
8. Ham C. Lost in Translation? Health Systems in the US and the UK. *Social Policy and Administration* 2005; **39**: 192–209.
9. National Audit Office. *Improving IT Procurement*. HC 877, Session 2003–04. Stationery Office, London, 2004.
10. Booth N. Sharing patient information electronically throughout the NHS. *British Medical Journal* 2003; **327**: 114–115.
11. Silverman D. *Doing Qualitative Research: A Practical Handbook*. SAGE, Thousand Oaks, CA, 2004.
12. Yin R. *Case Study Research: Design and Methods*, 3rd edn. SAGE, Newbury Park, CA, 2002.
13. Sheaff R, Marshall M, Rogers A, Roland M, Sibbald B & Pickard S. Governmentality by network in English primary healthcare. *Social Policy and Administration* 2004; **38**: 89–103.

14. Hammersley M & Atkinson P. *Ethnography: Principles in Practice*, 2nd edn. Routledge, London, 1995. Chapter 1.
15. Pawson R & Tilley N. *Realistic Evaluation*. SAGE, London, 1997. Chapter 3.
16. Silverman D. *Interpreting Qualitative Data*. SAGE, London, 1993. Chapter 7.

CHAPTER 11

Action research

Julienne Meyer

The barriers to the uptake of the findings of traditional quantitative biomedical research in clinical practice are increasingly being recognised [1,2]. Certain forms of qualitative research may make it easier for research to influence day-to-day practice. Action research is particularly suited to identifying problems in clinical practice and helping to develop potential solutions to improve practice [3], and is increasingly being employed in health-related settings. Although not synonymous with qualitative research, action research usually draws on qualitative methods and is frequently written up as a case study (see Chapter 10).

What is action research?

Like qualitative research in general, action research is not easily defined. It is a style of research rather than a specific method. It is a form of participatory research in which researchers work explicitly *with*, *for* and *by* people rather than undertake research *on* them [4]. It differs from other forms of participatory research in its focus on action. Its strength lies in its focus on generating solutions to practical problems and its ability to empower practitioners – getting them to engage with research and subsequent 'development' or implementation activities. Practitioners can be involved when they choose to research their own practice [5] or when an outside researcher is engaged to help them to identify problems, seek and implement potential solutions, and systematically monitor and reflect on the process and outcomes of change [6,7]. The level of interest in practitioner-led research is increasing in the United Kingdom, in part as a response to recent proposals to 'modernise' the National Health Service (NHS), for example, through the development of new forms of clinical governance [8] and other national initiatives (e.g. the NHS Research and Development Strategy, the Cochrane Collaboration, and Centres for Evidence Based Practice) which emphasise that research and development should be the business of every clinician. Waterman *et al.* [9: 11] define action research as

> a period of inquiry, which describes, interprets and explains social situations while executing a change intervention aimed at improvement and involvement. It is problem-focused, context-specific and future-oriented. Action research is a group activity with an explicit value basis and is founded on a partnership between action researchers and participants, all of whom are involved in the change process. The participatory process is educative and empowering, involving a dynamic approach in which problem identification, planning, action and evaluation are interlinked. Knowledge may be advanced through reflection and research, and qualitative and quantitative research methods may be employed to collect data. Different types of knowledge may be produced by action research, including practical and propositional. Theory may be generated and refined, and its general application explored through cycles of the action research process.

Most definitions incorporate three important elements, namely its participatory character, its democratic impulse, and its simultaneous contribution to both social science and social change [10].

Participation

Participation is fundamental to action research; it is an approach that demands that participants perceive the need to change and are willing to play an active role both in the research and change process. Whilst all research requires willing subjects, the level of commitment required in an action research study goes beyond simply agreeing to answer questions or to be observed. The clear-cut demarcation between 'researcher' and 'researched' found in other types of research may not be apparent in action research. The research design is *negotiated* with participants in a continuous process, making obtaining informed consent at the outset problematic. Action researchers, therefore, need to agree on an ethical code of practice with participants (Winter and Munn-Giddings offer some guidance on this [3]). Participation in the research and in the process of change can be threatening, and conflicts may arise – as a number of studies have shown [11,12]. For example, in one action research study [6], the process of asking for suggestions for improvements and feeding them back to participants had a profound effect on the dynamics of a multidisciplinary team. Not all participants in the study felt comfortable questioning their own practice and examining their own roles and responsibilities. Indeed, the nurse in charge found it particularly threatening and this resulted in her seeking employment elsewhere [13]. Where an outside researcher is working with practitioners it is important to obtain their trust and agree upon rules on the control of data and their use, and on how potential conflict will be resolved within the project. The way in which such rules are agreed upon demonstrates a second important feature of action research, namely its democratic impulse.

Democracy in action research

Action research is concerned with intervening to change and improve practice [14]. As such, it can be seen as a form of 'critical' social science [15]. This philosophical underpinning is a key difference between action research and other case study approaches. Democracy in action research usually requires participants to be seen as equals of the researcher. The researcher works as a facilitator of change, consulting with participants not only on the action process, but also on how it will be evaluated. One benefit of designing a study in conjunction with practitioners is that it can make the research process and outcomes more meaningful to practitioners, by rooting them in the reality of day-to-day practice.

Throughout the study, findings are fed back to participants for validation and to inform decisions about the next stage of the study. This formative style is responsive to events as they naturally occur and frequently entails 'collaborative spirals' of planning, acting, observing, reflecting and re-planning [16]. Figure 11.1 represents these spirals, showing smaller 'spin-off spirals' branching out from larger spirals of activity to illustrate that action research can address many different problems at one time without losing sight of the main issue.

However, as has already been noted, feeding back findings to participants can be, and often is, very threatening. Democratic practice is not always a feature of health care settings so care needs to be taken in such settings. An action researcher needs to be able to work across traditional boundaries (e.g. between professionals, between health and social care, and between hospital and community care) and juggle different, sometimes competing agendas. Other skills, in addition to research ability, are clearly of paramount importance

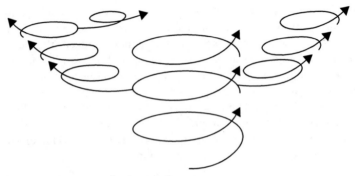

Figure 11.1 Action–reflection spirals.

in practice development, including cognitive, political, communicative, facilitative, clinical, visionary, motivational, empathic and experiential skills [17].

Contribution to social science and social change

The focus on change, and the level of involvement by participants in the research process, has led some to question the difference between action research and other management techniques such as continuous quality improvement [18]. Such criticisms are often founded on a fundamental misunderstanding of the nature of action research and its potential contribution. Some researchers argue that action research is more informative locally than globally [18], but this misrepresents the potential of generalisation from case study research [19]. Moreover, action research can provide a way of dealing with the numerous factors that influence the implementation of evidence into practice [20] by developing knowledge more appropriate to day-to-day practice [4,9].

In considering the contribution of action research to knowledge, it is important to note that generalisations made from action research studies differ from those made on the basis of more conventional forms of research. To some extent, reports of action research studies rely on the reader to underwrite the account of the research by drawing on their own knowledge of human situations. It is, therefore, important, when reporting action research, to describe the work in its rich contextual detail. The onus is on the researcher to make his/her own values and beliefs explicit in the research account so that any bias is evident. This can be facilitated by writing self-reflective fieldnotes during the research. According to Carr and Kemmis [10], a successful report can be characterised by 'the shock of recognition' – the quality of the account that enables readers to assess its relevance to themselves and their own practice situations. Feeding back findings throughout the action research study makes it possible to check the accuracy of the account with participants. However, interpreting the relevance of the findings to other practice situations ultimately rests with the reader, unless theoretical generalisation is claimed.

Given that change is problematic, the success of action research should not be judged solely in terms of the size of change achieved or the immediate implementation of solutions. Instead, success can often be viewed in relation to what has been learnt from the experience of undertaking the work. For instance, a study that set out to explore the issues arising from the introduction of a new role (that of interprofessional care co-ordinator) [21] did not result in achieving all the changes identified as needed in the course of the study. However, the lessons learnt from the research were reviewed in the context of national policy and research, and fed back to those working in the organisation and, as a result, changes were subsequently made within the organisation based on the study's recommendations.

Different types of action research

There are many different types of action research. Hart and Bond [22] suggest that there are some key characteristics, which not only distinguish action research from other methods, but which also determine the range of approaches to action research. They present a typology of action research identifying four basic types: experimental, organisational, professionalizing and empowering. Whilst this typology is useful in understanding the wide range of action research, its multi-dimensional nature means that it is not particularly easy to classify individual studies. Instead this typology may be better used as a framework for critiquing individual studies [23]. Somekh notes that different occupational cultures can affect action research and for this reason, suggests [24] that action research should be grounded in the values and discourse of the individual or group rather than rigidly adhering to a particular methodological perspective.

Action research in health care

Because action research focuses on change it is seen as a useful framework for researching innovation, alongside realistic evaluation [25,26]. Elsewhere, interest in action research within health care settings has been demonstrated by the commissioning of a systematic review of action research by the English Department of Health Technology Assessment R&D programme [9]. This review identified 59 studies (72 reports) published between January 1975 and July 1998, and these are usefully summarised in the final report.

Ong [27] advocates the value of action research within health care settings on the basis of changes in the requirements of health care management and policy. She highlights the need for new, systematic approaches to encouraging user participation in health services. She suggests that 'Rapid Appraisal' is an ideal method for engaging users in the development of health care policy and practice. Rapid Appraisal is a type of action research, hitherto predominantly used in developing countries, which focuses on participatory methods to foster change, using ideas derived from the field of community development. Her book [28] gives excellent detail not only on the philosophical and theoretical underpinnings of Rapid Appraisal, but also on how such studies should be conducted.

Action research has also been used in hospital rather than wider community settings to facilitate closer partnerships between staff and users. In a study that focused on the introduction of lay participation in care within a general medical ward of a London teaching hospital, the action researcher worked for one year in a multidisciplinary team (see Box 11.1) [6]. In the course of the study, it emerged that to foster closer partnerships with users and carers, professionals needed to change their practice to work more collaboratively with one another. As a result, three main action–reflection spirals emerged in the project: reorganising the work of the ward; improving multidisciplinary communication; and increasing lay participation in care. Each action–reflection spiral generated related activities, known as spin-off spirals. For instance, stemming from the main lay participation in care action-reflection spiral, a spin-off spiral focused on the medical staff teaching patients more about their treatments.

A range of research methods was used, including depth interviews, questionnaires, documentary analysis and participant observation. Throughout the study, preliminary findings were fed back to

Box 11.1 Lay participation in care: an action research study
[6,29,30]

Participation	Careful negotiation to recruit willing volunteers to examine practice and initiate lay participation in care 'Bottom-up' approach to change via weekly team meetings Researcher as facilitator and multidisciplinary team member
Democracy	Goal of empowering practitioners and lay people in this setting Working collaboratively with multidisciplinary teams Participants given 'ownership' of the data to determine how it might be shared with a wider audience
Contribution to social science and social change	Findings constantly fed back to practitioners, leading to changes (such as, improvements in interprofessional working) Dissemination of findings of local and national relevance
Evaluation methods	Case study of multidisciplinary team on one general medical ward in a London teaching hospital using: • qualitative methods to highlight key themes emerging in the project • quantitative methods for comparison of sub groups
Main action–reflection spirals	Reorganising the work of the ward • Changes in patient care planning • New reporting system, including bedside handover with patient • Introduction of modified form of primary nursing system Multidisciplinary communication. Weekly team meetings instituted • Introduction of a handout for new staff and team communication sheet. Closer liaison with community nurses before discharge

> **Box 11.1** Continued
>
> Lay participation in care
> • Development of resources for patient health education
> • Introduction of medicine reminder card system
> • Patient information leaflet inviting patients to participate in care
>
> Results   Insights into health professionals' perceptions of lay participation in care
> Some positive changes achieved (e.g. improved attitudes to lay participation in care, patient education, improved ward organisation)
> Identified barriers to changing health care practice

participants through weekly team meetings to help guide the project. Whilst positive change was demonstrated over time, the analysis generated two main data sets on the health professionals' perceptions of lay participation in care and the difficulties encountered in changing practice [29,30].

The value of using qualitative methods and an action research approach can best be demonstrated from this example in relation to the data on the health professionals' perceptions of lay participation in care. Qualitative methods were used alongside quantitative methods such as attitudinal scales and self-administered questionnaires as part of a process of triangulation (see Chapters 8 and 9 for more on this). Qualitative methods can be useful in reinterpreting the findings from more quantitative methods. In this study, health professionals expressed extremely positive views about user and carer involvement when completing an attitude scale [31]. However, further research suggested that they had some serious doubts and concerns and that these were inhibiting the implementation of lay participation. Previous research on health professionals' attitudes towards user and carer involvement had tended to rely solely on structured instruments and had found that health professionals held generally positive attitudes towards it [32–34]. By contrast, using mixed methods, it was possible to explore the relationship between attitudes and practices, and to explain what happened when lay participation was introduced into a practice setting. Findings suggested that, while policy documents were advocating lay participation in care, some health professionals were merely paying lip service to the concept and were also inadequately prepared to deliver it in practice. In addition, findings indicated that health professionals needed to learn to collaborate more closely with each other, by developing a common understanding and approach to patient care, to offer closer partnerships with users and carers. Whilst one should not over-generalise from a single case study, this research led to serious questioning of the value of previous quantitative research, which had suggested that health professionals held positive attitudes towards lay participation in care. By using action research and working closely with practitioners to explore issues in a practical context, more insight was gained into how the rhetoric of policy might be better translated into reality.

Conclusion

Action research does not focus exclusively on user and carer involvement, though clearly its participatory principles make it an obvious choice of research method to explore these issues. It can be used more widely, for example, to foster better practice across interprofessional boundaries and between different health care settings [21,35]. Action research can also be used by clinicians to research their own practice [16]. It is an eclectic approach to research, which draws on a variety of data collection methods. However, its focus on the process as well as the outcomes of change helps to explain the frequent use of qualitative methods by action researchers.

Further reading

Reason P & Bradbury H. *Handbook of Action Research: Participative Inquiry and Practice*. SAGE, London, 2001.

Waterman H, Tillen D, Dickson R & de Koning K. *Action research: a systematic review and guidance for assessment*. Health Technology Assessment 2001; **5**(23).

References

1. Strauss SE, Richardson WS, Glasziou P & Haynes RB. *Evidence-Based Medicine: How to Practise and Teach EBM*, 3rd edn. Churchill Livingstone, Edinburgh, 2005.
2. Trinder L & Reynolds S. *Evidence-Based Practice: A Critical Appraisal*. Blackwell Science Ltd, Oxford, 2000.

3. Winter R & Munn-Giddings C. *A Handbook for Action Research in Health and Social Care*. Routledge, London, 2001.

4. Reason P & Bradbury H. *Handbook of Action Research. Participative Inquiry and Practice*. SAGE, London, 2001.

5. Rolfe G. *Expanding Nursing Knowledge: Understanding and Researching Your Own Practice*. Butterworth Heineman, Oxford, 1998.

6. Meyer JE. Lay participation in care in a hospital setting: an action research study. Nursing Praxis International, Portsmouth, 2001.

7. Titchen A & McGinley M. Facilitating practitioner research through critical companionship. *NTResearch* 2003; **8**:2:115–131.

8. Secretary of State for Health. *The New NHS: Modern, Dependable*. Cm 3807. The Stationery Office, London, 1997.

9. Waterman H, Tillen D, Dickson R *et al*. Action research: a systematic review and guidance for assessment. *Health Technology Assessment* 2001; **5**(23).

10. Carr W & Kemmis S. Becoming critical: education, knowledge and action research. Falmer Press, London, 1986.

11. Waterson J. Balancing research and action: reflections on an action research project in a social services department. *Social Policy and Administration*. 2000; **34**: 494–508.

12. Ashburner C, Meyer J, Johnson B *et al*. Using action research to address loss of personhood in a continuing care setting. *Illness, Crisis and Loss* 2004; **12**:4: 23–37.

13. Meyer JE. New paradigm research in practice: the trials and tribulations of action research. *Journal of Advanced Nursing* 1993; **18**: 1066–1072.

14. Coghlan D & Brannick T. *Doing Action Research in Your Own Organisation*. SAGE, London, 2001.

15. Brown T & Jones L. *Action Research and Postmodernism: Congruence and Critique*. Open University Press, Buckingham, 2001.

16. McNiff J. *Action Research: Principles and Practice*. Macmillan Education Ltd, London, 1988.

17. McCormack B & Garbett R. The characteristics, qualities and skills of practice developers. *Journal of Clinical Nursing*, 2003; **12**: 317–325.

18. Lilford R, Warren R & Braunholtz D. Action research: a way of researching or a way of managing? [Journal Article] *Journal of Health Services & Research Policy* 2003; **8**:2: 100–104.

19. Sharp K. The case for case studies in nursing research: the problem of generalisation. *Journal of Advanced Nursing*, 1998; **27**: 785–789.

20. Rycroft-Malone J, Harvey G, Seers K *et al*. An exploration of the factors that influence the implementation of evidence into practice. *Journal of Clinical Nursing* 2004; **13**:913–924.

21. Bridges J, Meyer J, Glynn M *et al*. Interprofessional care co-ordinator: the benefits and tensions associated with a new role in U.K. acute health care. *International Journal of Nursing Studies* 2003; **40**: 599–607.

22. Hart E & Bond M. Action research for health and social care. A guide to practice. Open University Press, Buckingham, 1995.

23. Lyon J. Applying Hart and Bond's typology; implementing clinical supervision in an acute setting. *Nurse Researcher* 1999; **6**: 39–53.

24. Somekh B. Inhabiting each other's castles: towards knowledge and mutual growth though collaboration. *Educational Action Research Journal* 1994; **2**(3): 357–381.

25. Greenhalgh T, Robert G, Bate P *et al.* How to Spread Good Ideas. A systematic review of the literature on diffusion, dissemination and sustainability of innovations in health service delivery and organization. Report for the National Co-ordinating Centre for NHS Service Delivery and Organisation R & D (NCCSDO). London School of Hygiene and Tropical Medicine, London, April 2004.

26. Pawson R & Tilley N. *Realistic Evaluation.* SAGE, London, 1997.

27. Ong BN. *The Practice of Health Services Research.* Chapman & Hall, London, 1993: 65–82.

28. Ong BN. *Rapid Appraisal and Health Policy.* Chapman & Hall, 1996.

29. Meyer JE. Lay participation in care: a challenge for multi-disciplinary teamwork. *Journal of Interprofessional Care* 1993; **7**: 57–66.

30. Meyer JE. Lay participation in care: threat to the status quo. In: Wilson-Barnett J & Macleod Clark J, eds. *Research in Health Promotion and Nursing.* Macmillan, London, 1993: 86–100.

31. Brooking J. Patient and family participation in nursing care: the development of a nursing process measuring scale. University of London, London, unpublished PhD thesis, 1986.

32. Pankratz L & Pankratz D. Nursing autonomy and patients' rights: development of a nursing attitude scale. *Journal of Health and Social Behavior* 1974; **15**: 211–216.

33. Citron MJ. Attitudes of nurses regarding the patients' role in the decision-making process and their implications for nursing education. *Dissertation Abstracts International* 1978; **38**: 584.

34. Linn LS & Lewis CE. Attitudes towards self-care amongst practising physicians. *Medical Care* 1979; **17**: 183–190.

35. Meyer J & Bridges J. An action research study into the organisation of care of older people in the accident and emergency department. City University, London, 1998.

CHAPTER 12

Consensus development methods

Nick Black

Consensus development methods are not typically considered among qualitative methods as they involve scaling, questionnaires and quantitative methods of analysis. Despite this, they are included in this book as an example of a technique that organises qualitative judgements and, which is concerned to understand the meanings that people use when making decisions about health care.

Why use consensus development methods?

Many key decisions in health care have to be made without adequate objective information. Such decisions range from how best to treat patients, what services to provide, how best to organise and deliver services, what research should be prioritised and *horizon-scanning* (forecasting the future). Decision-making in the face of uncertainty is a common challenge for clinicians, managers and policy-makers. One traditional solution is for a powerful individual or someone deemed to be best equipped for the task to make the decision. However, it is generally agreed that there are advantages in a group rather than an individual making decisions: groups bring a wider range of knowledge and experience; interaction between group members both stimulates consideration of more options and challenges received ideas; idiosyncrasies are filtered out; and a group view may carry more weight than that of any one individual [1].

Traditionally, group decision-making has relied on an informal approach, such as a committee. Indeed, this remains the principal approach in most walks of life despite several long-standing and widely observed shortcomings: domination by particular individuals; pressures to agree with the majority or the view of powerful people; more extreme decisions than any single individual would advocate; and complex issues remaining unresolved.

Since the 1950s, formal approaches to decision-making have been developed and increasingly used in many areas, including health care. Their advantages over informal approaches are that a transparent structured method can eliminate the negative aspects mentioned above and provide scientific credibility. In health care, these methods have been used for three main purposes: the development of clinical and organisational guidelines; determining priorities as to which services to provide, what topics to research, and which outcomes to measure; and drawing up criteria by which policy issues (e.g. research quality, methods of paying for health care, etc.) can be judged.

In essence, consensus development methods attempt to identify all the issues that are relevant, then to frame those issues in the form of explicit statements and finally to obtain a group's view as to their level of agreement with each statement by means of a *Likert scale* (a measure of agreement typically on a 5- or 9-point scale ranging from strong to weak agreement). In this way, unstructured qualitative discussion is converted into structured quantitative recording of views in an explicit, transparent way.

Which methods exist?

The key features of formal consensus development methods are:
- provision of independent evidence – group members are provided with a synthesis of all available scientific or research evidence, produced using rigorous methods;
- privacy – individual members of a group express their views in private such that the other members remain unaware of each person's judgment;
- opportunity for individuals to change their views in the light of seeing the anonymised initial views of all group members (and, with a nominal group, hearing explanations for differences in views); and
- explicit and transparent derivation of the group's decision, based on pre-arranged statistical methods of aggregation and analysis.

Three methods of developing group consensus have been used in health care though one, consensus development conferences, has largely been abandoned and is not discussed further here. The other two are nominal group techniques and Delphi surveys. Although each has some core features, each can be modified and implemented in a variety of ways.

Nominal group techniques (NGTs)

These are so named because the group's view is derived from the aggregation of individual members' views rather than from the group arriving at a communal view. The group usually comprises 8–12 members. Any fewer and the reliability of the group view would be in jeopardy [2], any more and group discussions would prove unmanageable and frustrating for participants.

There are usually three stages. First, the members are asked to suggest (in writing) what the key relevant issues are concerning the topic (e.g. in developing guidelines on indications for a hip replacement, people might suggest the patient's age or degree of hip pain as highly relevant). All the suggestions are then aggregated by the person organising the process. Second, a structured questionnaire covering all the issues (and combinations of issues) is produced and each group member is asked to rate their level of agreement with each suggestion on a Likert scale (e.g. 'people aged 65–74 years with mild pain should have hip replacements'). Third, the aggregated responses, showing the distribution of members' views, are returned to the participants who meet to discuss areas of disagreement. The discussion is facilitated by a non-participant. Following the discussion, members rate their level of agreement again, whether or not their view has changed in the light of their knowledge of others' views and explanations. Although this stage can be repeated, in practice, group views show little or no further change. The group views are then analysed according to pre-arranged definitions of agreement and disagreement.

One of the most frequently used versions of NGTs in the health sector was developed by UCLA/RAND in which the first two stages are conducted by mail and the group only meets for the third stage [3]. This clearly has practical advantages over a process requiring three meetings.

Delphi surveys

The main limitation of NGTs is the relatively small number of people who can participate (because of the practicalities of facilitating a meeting) and the requirements of getting all the participants together for at least one meeting. Not surprisingly, people have questioned the representativeness of nominal group views. The alternative approach, a Delphi survey, avoids these limitations. There is no practical limit to the number of participants, though there is little to be gained methodologically from including more than about 50 people. However, to gain greater 'ownership' of the decision that emerges, it may be politically necessary to include a larger number of those who form the target audience for the output.

The process only differs from an NGT in one major respect – the group of participants never meets. Everything is done by mail. This means that a much more geographically dispersed sample can participate. The potential disadvantage is that the participants do not get to hear the reasons for any divergent views (though participants could be asked to explain their views and these could be communicated in writing during the second round). The basis of any change to their initial ratings is, therefore, purely their response to being made aware of the views of fellow participants. As a result, the extent of agreement or consensus is less than that achieved with nominal groups [4]. This has to be balanced by the greater reliability of Delphi surveys, though this is due entirely to the larger size of the groups.

Practical issues

Selection of participants

Given the purpose of the exercise is to make decisions that will be well-received and have an impact on existing policy or practice, the key issue when selecting participants is that they represent the target audience for the output. So, it makes little sense to seek just the views of general practitioners if the target audience is community nurses. In practice, given the multi-professional or multidisciplinary nature of most health care activities, it is advisable to ensure that all relevant professional or stakeholder groups or 'tribes' are represented. It may well be that patients or their lay carers should also be included.

The greatest concern people have about NGTs stems from the small size of the groups. How can around ten participants be representative? Within defined specialist or professional categories, studies have shown that the particular individuals selected have little impact on the decision (i.e. any ten community nurses will come to similar decisions) [5]. What does make a difference is participants 'expertise'. Ten community nurses are likely to make different decisions from ten general practitioners or ten patients. Participants tend to view those activities with which they are most familiar more favourably than participants who are not so familiar. For example, cardiac surgeons are more likely than cardiologists or community nurses to view surgery as the correct treatment for a patient. Equally, cardiologists may advocate medical treatment and community nurses may favour lifestyle changes.

Another frequently voiced concern is that the less specialised members of a group (most notably, patients or lay people) cannot contribute much and should be excluded, leaving the decision-making to those with the most specialised knowledge. In practice, the knowledge and ability of lay people is often underestimated by specialists. In addition, while the highly technical aspects of the topic may be beyond the understanding of some people, other aspects such as social, economic and ethical implications, may not be. Indeed, disagreements within heterogeneous groups may be based on differing values rather than differences in interpreting complex scientific information. It is important that such disagreements are addressed if the resulting decisions are to be widely accepted.

Group meetings

A review of research-based information should be provided to all participants and they should be encouraged to read it and bring it with them to nominal group meetings to refer to when necessary. The only study to look at the impact of providing a review to nominal groups found that their decisions were more likely to be consistent with the research evidence than if no review was provided [6]. It seems likely that the more user-friendly the presentation of the research evidence, the more likely it is that participants will assimilate it.

For most participants in a nominal group, it will be a new experience. Unlike informal group meetings, participants need to pay constant attention and engage with all items under discussion. It is a pressurised and demanding exercise that has to be carefully managed by the facilitator. Handled well, it is also a rewarding experience that most participants enjoy and value. It makes sense to treat the participants well. It is well worth making the people feel their participation is appreciated by holding the meeting in a quiet, comfortable setting and provide good quality sustenance. Generally, discussion sessions should last no longer than two hours and ideally there should be only two sessions in a day.

It is important that the person running the meeting acts as a facilitator and not a chairperson. That is easier if the person has little knowledge of, or views on, the topic being discussed. The facilitator's role is to explain the process, stressing that participants should not change their views just to enable the group to reach consensus. Participants should, however, listen and consider other members' views in an open and respectful way. Another task for the facilitator is to ensure that all members of the group get a fair chance to contribute. The less powerful tend to be less assertive and need some encouragement to participate. But perhaps the most important task is to ensure the group covers all aspects of the topic. It is no good if at the end of the process only half the issues have been discussed and rated. It is necessary for the facilitator to allow sufficient time for discussion, but not let the group devote too much time to any particular issue. This requires sensitive judgment and being prepared to stop discussions and move the group on.

As with focus groups (see Chapter 3), it is not possible for the facilitator also to make a record of the salient points in the discussion. So it is necessary to have an observer taking notes and for the discussion to be audio-taped. Groups should be reassured that any use of the recording will not reveal individuals' identity, even if verbatim quotes are extracted.

Analysis

Analysing the quantitative output from consensus development methods is an evolving science. New ways are frequently being explored and reported. However, despite the range of methods available, they all share the same goals: determination of the group's view (some measure of central tendency); and the extent of agreement within the group (a measure of dispersal). Given that group views are rarely normally distributed, the median rather than the mean score should be used for the former. An appropriate measure of dispersal is the inter-quartile range, although other options exist.

For those statements for which the group managed to reach a consensus (i.e. individuals' ratings were sufficiently narrowly distributed), it is necessary to translate a quantitative score (a median) into a qualitative judgement (agreement with the statement; disagreement with the statement; neither). Generally, Likert rating scales are divided into thirds so that the lowest scores indicate dis-agreement, the highest scores signify agreement, and those in the central third show that the group is equivocal. For example, if a 9-point scale has been used, any medians lying between 1 and 3 are deemed to indicate disagreement with the statement.

As may be apparent, a critical factor in the analysis is how strict a definition of consensus is used. At one extreme, if all group members were required to give exactly the same score, consensus would be reached on very few statements. At the other extreme, if a wide distribution of scores was accepted, consensus could be achieved for most statements. One commonly adopted rule has been that on a 9-point scale, all the ratings must lie within a 3-point range to constitute consensus. Whatever rules are adopted, they should be decided beforehand and not after the data have been collected and analysed.

One potential hazard is that one or more members of a group decide to disrupt the process by deliberately providing extreme rat-ings out of line with the rest of the group. This could result in no consensus being achieved for any statement. To guard against this, it is common practice to decide in advance that one or more outlier scorer for each statement will be excluded. The number excluded will depend partly on the group size. With a group of 10, it would be acceptable to exclude one or two.

The impact that rules can have on outcomes can be seen in Table 12.1 in which both the above aspects are explored. Use of relaxed definitions of agreement (all ratings within any 3-point range) compared with a strict definition (all ratings within pre-defined 3-point ranges such as 1–3) had little impact on the pro-portion of statements reaching agreement. In contrast, excluding some outliers greatly increased the groups' levels of agreement.

A new modified approach

Given some of the limitations that have been described, there is a case for a new approach. Apart from any methodological limitations, the existing methods tend to have become rather cumbersome and expensive in some organizations' hands. The development of clin-ical and organisational guidelines by National Institute for Health and Clinical Excellence (NICE) in England often involves up to 20 meetings of a group over 1–2 years, an approach that is not

Table 12.1 Impact of different definitions of agreement on the proportion of statements for which nominal groups reached consensus

Topic	Include all ratings		Exclude furthest ratings*	
	Strict	Relaxed	Strict	Relaxed
Coronary angiography [7]	28	29		
Endoscopy [7]	25	25		
Carotid endarterectomy [7]	41	41		
Cholecystectomy [8]				
– mixed group	45	47	63	67
– surgical group	35	35	57	61
Total hip replacement [9]				
– UK	42	42	53	59
– Japan	23	32	50	69

Strict = all individual ratings in 1–3, 4–6 or 7–9 bands; relaxed = all individual ratings in any 3-point band.
* exclusion of the two ratings furthest from the median.

sustainable. So there is also a need for a quicker, more efficient approach.

One alternative model has recently been proposed [10]. It involves only three nominal group meetings. At the first meeting the group identifies the specific aspects of the topic to be examined. Methodologists then review and synthesise the research evidence and other relevant material, taking care to document any judgements about conflicting evidence and methodological limitations of the evidence. This material and the group members' views are then used to develop and pilot a questionnaire.

Members of the group are then mailed the literature review and the questionnaire to be completed in private. The group's view is presented at the second meeting where areas of disagreement can be explored. Participants then have the opportunity to revise their ratings privately. Notes are taken during the meeting and it is audio-taped to enable a thematic analysis of the influence issues such as cost, effectiveness, priority, feasibility and acceptability have on the ratings. The representativeness of the group's view can then be checked by mailing a random sample of the items covered in the questionnaire to a large, similarly composed group.

Based on the nominal group's views (modified if it is shown in the survey to be unrepresentative), the questionnaire results can be turned into qualitative decisions or recommendations. These are then mailed to the nominal group members who reassemble to discuss the draft decisions at a third and final meeting. The published output includes an indication of the underlying assumptions of the group and the strength of support for each recommendation together with the extent of agreement within the group on each statement.

Conclusions

Although the heart of formal consensus development methods is a quantitative approach, their purpose is to organise and make sense of qualitative data (i.e. peoples' diverse opinions and judgments). Traditionally, the complexity of multiple views was consigned to the 'black box' of informal groups that tended to perpetuate existing views and power structures. Challenges were difficult to mount as it was unclear how decisions had been arrived at. With formal methods, group decision-making is exposed, and thus made more accountable and democratic.

Further reading

Murphy MK, Black NA, Lamping DL *et al.* Consensus development methods, and their use in clinical guideline development. *Health Technology Assessment* 1998; **2**(3): 1–88.

References

1. Murphy MK, Black NA, Lamping DL *et al.* Consensus development methods, and their use in clinical guideline development. *Health Technology Assessment* 1998; **2**(3): 1–88.
2. Richardson FM. Peer review of medical care. *Medical Care* 1972; **10**: 29–39.
3. Fitch K, Bernstein SJ, Aguilar MD *et al. The RAND/UCLA Appropriateness Method User's Manual.* RAND, Santa Monica, CA, 2001.
4. Hutchings A, Raine R, Sanderson C *et al.* A comparison of formal consensus methods used for developing clinical guidelines. *Journal of Health Services Research & Policy* (in press).

5. Hutchings A & Raine R. A systematic review of factors affecting the judgements produced by formal consensus development methods in health care. *Journal of Health Services Research & Policy* (in press).

6. Raine R, Sanderson C, Hutchings A *et al.* An experimental study of determinants of group judgments in clinical guideline development. *Lancet* 2004; **364**: 429–437.

7. Park RE, Fink A, Brook RH *et al.* Physician ratings of appropriate indications for three procedures: theoretical indications versus indications used in practice. *American Journal of Public Health* 1989; **79**: 445–447.

8. Scott EA & Black N. Appropriateness of cholecystectomy in the UK – a consensus panel approach. *Gut* 1991; **32**: 1066–1070.

9. Imamura K, Gair R, McKee CM *et al.* Appropriateness of total hip replacement in the UK. *World Hospitals & Health Services* 1997; **32**: 10–14.

10. Raine R, Sanderson C & Black N. Developing clinical guidelines: a challenge to current methods. *British Medical Journal* 2005; **331**: 631–633.

CHAPTER 13

Synthesising qualitative research

Catherine Pope, Nicholas Mays

Introduction

Qualitative research is, by its very nature, often focused on individual cases such as a single setting or a specific group of patients or health care practitioners. Even larger scale qualitative pieces of work – such as studies involving relatively large numbers of interviews or multiple settings – often focus on the minutiae of everyday life and provide detail about a unique local context and moment in time. As other chapters in this book attest, this kind of rich description is one of the strengths of qualitative research. However, one of the drawbacks is that this can produce fascinating, insightful, but hard-to-generalise studies. Even when it is possible to find a group of such studies on a similar topic and carried out in comparable settings or with similar respondents, the highly specific nature of the research can make it difficult to grasp the cumulative message from such a body of evidence. This can pose problems for those wishing to use the findings of qualitative research – for example, to inform policy-making or decisions about health care provision. Questions that might be asked are: what do a set of studies conducted in different countries about specific health care reforms and innovations tell us about how organisational change in general happens in health systems? Or, what do the individual studies of patients' attitudes to taking medicines tell us about the patient experience of medicine-taking overall?

One way of attempting to answer these kinds of questions might be to conduct a narrative review of literature, perhaps identifying key themes from each of the studies included. However, while such reviews can aggregate papers, such literature reviews do not necessarily *integrate* evidence or develop new cumulative knowledge. In quantitative health research, systematic reviewing techniques have been developed, such as meta-analysis, to pool the results of randomised controlled trials [1], which enable the integration and appraisal of quantitative evidence. These approaches have become standardised with the aims of ensuring that the process is adequately documented and that the findings are valid and reliable, as far as possible. Systematic reviews can also encompass non-experimental research findings, though in these cases it is seldom possible to pool the data from studies with different designs. Systematic reviews have tended to include only quantitative findings, but recently there have been attempts to include qualitative research in systematic reviews, where relevant [2,3].

Alongside the development of largely quantitative systematic review methods, researchers have also begun to explore methods that allow the integration or *synthesis* of qualitative research evidence. Methods for synthesising qualitative research evidence are evolving and some are less well developed than others. This chapter looks at some of the methods of synthesis that are currently being developed and applied to qualitative research in the health field.

Should we synthesise at all?

There are arguments about whether it is feasible or desirable to synthesise evidence from multiple research studies, just as there are arguments about whether it is legitimate to mix different qualitative, and qualitative and quantitative methods in a single primary research study (see Chapter 9 on mixed methods). Some contend that aggregation destroys the integrity of individual studies and that differences in theoretical outlook and method fundamentally militate against synthesis. This position was discussed in Chapter 8 on the assessment of the quality of qualitative research. For those who hold that each qualitative study is a unique representation of multiple realities or truths the idea of synthesising several studies is anathema. However, as we made clear in Chapter 8, we adopt a 'subtle realist' position [4] that holds that there is ultimately an underlying social reality that research studies attempt in different ways to describe. Moreover, as applied researchers working in health care research and policy environments, we believe that a significant proportion of research should be directed towards answering questions and supporting decision-making relevant to health services and policy. We are also conscious that much health care research is not cumulative and does not build on work undertaken before. Even with the rise of electronic search engines and information techno-logy, studies frequently do not reference or discuss other comparable research in the same field [5]. In addition, qualitative research reports can be difficult to locate [6–8]. For all these reasons synthesis is a desirable and increasingly important part of qualitative health research.

The purpose of synthesis

Synthesis can be conducted for different purposes. It may help to identify gaps in knowledge or areas for further research. It can be conducted to summarise the implications of the qualitative evidence as part of a broader review process that includes a systematic review or other analyses of quantitative evidence. Or, it may aim directly to inform decision-making. As a result there are many different audi-ences for synthesis. These can include other researchers, health care practitioners or providers of services, managers, policy makers and research funders. In addition to attending to the purpose of the syn-thesis, it is worth recognising that these different audiences may have different needs in terms of how the synthesis is conducted and expressed.

Methods for synthesising qualitative research

This chapter considers three of the main methods that can be used to synthesise qualitative research: narrative synthesis, cross-case ana-lysis and meta-ethnography. Before describing these methods, there are some preliminary considerations that apply to any review or synthesis.

Although this may not always be possible at the outset, it is important to specify the question(s) underpinning the synthesis. Sometimes questions are adapted or re-framed during the process of collecting and analysing the evidence, but as with other aspects of qualitative research it is important to be clear ultimately about the question(s) addressed. Preliminary scoping of potential literat-ure sources can help the process of refining the question(s) prior to a more extensive search. The strategy for searching and decisions about which literature to include are partly dependent on the size of the literature, and if there happen to be a large number of relev-ant studies it may be necessary to consider some form of sampling.

Electronic searching for qualitative literature can be particularly difficult as some databases do not use appropriate index terms. For this reason hand searching of journals is strongly advised alongside consulting subject area experts. It is worth remembering that much qualitative literature is published in monographs, book chapters or theses, as well as journal papers. In contrast to some systematic reviews, qualitative synthesises can cover long time periods, partly to ensure that early 'classic' studies that may make a significant theoretical contribution are included [9].

There is some debate as to the worth of appraising the literature for quality with a view to excluding certain studies before undertaking the synthesis of findings [5,8]. Some authors argue that this should not be done, even though it is a common feature of quantitative systematic reviews and, claim instead, that the value of specific pieces of research will only become apparent during the synthesis process. Thus 'weaker' papers can be included in qualitative syntheses as long as their relative quality is clear. As noted in Chapter 8, there are various checklists and guidelines for assessing research quality, some of which have been devised for use with qualitative synthesis. Such appraisal can be helpful in ensuring that the researchers conducting the synthesis are familiar with the strengths and weaknesses of each of the studies collected for the synthesis, but there does not seem to be compelling evidence that the results of such appraisal should be the only arbiter of inclusion.

Narrative synthesis
Narrative synthesis is rooted in a narrative or story-telling approach and seeks to generate new insights or knowledge by systematically and transparently bringing together existing research findings. Narrative synthesis aims to move beyond the kinds of traditional narrative literature reviews which summarize one study after another with little attempt at integration. In the United Kingdom, an Economic and Social Research Council (ESRC) funded project has developed helpful guidance for undertaking narrative synthesis [10] including worked applications of this approach. In essence, narrative syntheses entail the identification of key themes arising in the literature identified and the development of a narrative or 'story' that encompasses these. *Meta-narrative mapping* [11] (also called *realist synthesis*) is a specific form of narrative synthesis that has recently been developed. In meta-narrative mapping, the focus is on drawing out the central theories or causal mechanisms identified within

multiple studies and building an explanation of the body of research by telling the story of the evolution of the field of enquiry or mapping the domains covered by the literature in an area. In a meta-narrative mapping of the large, diverse literature on innovation in health care and other organisations, the resulting synthesis identified thirteen different research traditions and seven key dimensions relating to spread and sustainability of innovation and change. The authors were able to put these disparate elements together in a narrative structure, both chronologically and thematically (i.e. describing the theoretical development from early and more recent literature, and identifying thematic groupings) to tell the story of this extensive but complex literature.

Cross-case analysis
Qualitative cross-case analysis presents the findings from multiple cases (i.e. different studies) to develop new explanations for an entire body of findings. This typically uses some form of matrix display such as those advocated by Miles and Huberman [12]. Although developed for analysing primary qualitative data from a number of case studies, the same tabular ways of representing data can be used to explore and compare relationships between the findings of different studies. Matrices or charts are used to display variables, themes or concepts from a series of studies to facilitate systematic comparison. Yin [13] describes this process as akin to the constant comparative approach, as used in 'grounded theory' (see Chapters 1 and 7 for more on 'grounded theory'). He suggests using pattern matching (i.e. searching for similar variables) to group together key concepts with the aim of identifying the core or essential elements and thereby developing new concepts or explanations from the findings of a set of studies.

Meta-ethnography
Meta-ethnography [14] uses qualitative research techniques to re-analyse multiple qualitative reports. The name is slightly misleading in that it implies, wrongly, that the approach can only be used with ethnographic studies. It also unfortunately engenders some confusion with the term meta-analysis. A helpful worked example of this approach is provided by Britten *et al.* [15]. It involves induction and interpretation (i.e. re-analysis) or the published reports of previous studies. A key feature of meta-ethnography is the use of *reciprocal translation* – a process in which different studies are translated or interpreted into one another. This entails systematically searching

through each study, extracting key findings and interpretations, and comparing them with each other to develop a set of overarching concepts or overlapping areas. This process resembles the constant comparison methods used in primary qualitative research approaches such as 'grounded theory'. Each finding (e.g. a concept or interpretation) is examined to see how it is like (or unlike) those in the other studies, and these are matched, merged and adapted to enable the generation of a new, combined set of interpretations. The product of a meta-ethnography may be simply this reciprocal translation, but more often this can be developed further into a new *line of argument* synthesis. The originators of the approach [14] also suggest that it is possible to use meta-ethnography to demonstrate and explain opposing or refutational interpretations in the literature. An example of a 'line of argument' synthesis is provided by Pound *et al.*'s [5] meta-ethnography of published literature reporting patients' views of taking medicines prescribed for short- or long-term conditions. This identified seven main groups of papers related to corresponding groups of medicines/conditions and used this body of evidence to develop a new model of medicine taking and to expound the novel concept of patient *resistance* to medicines. The idea of 'resistance' is that patients actively engage with medicines – they deliberately modify and adapt their prescribed medication taking because of complex understandings, meanings and beliefs that they bring to medicine taking. According to this argument, non-compliance or non-adherence with regimens is not simply the result of a passive failure to take medicines, but is the result of active decision-making by the patient.

Synthesis of qualitative and quantitative evidence

As mentioned in Chapter 9, there is some controversy about whether we can or should combine qualitative and quantitative methods in primary studies, and these concerns are writ large whenever the subject of integrating qualitative and quantitative evidence from more than one study is mooted. We have argued elsewhere [16] that qualitative–quantitative synthesis is the logical extension of a mixed-method approach to research and one that offers considerable benefit to policy and health care decision-making. However, there is no single, agreed framework for synthesizing these diverse forms of evidence. There are four broad approaches potentially applicable for synthesising qualitative and quantitative research, which for simplicity, can be distinguished as narrative, qualitative, quantitative and Bayesian. In the context of policy and health care decision-making, Bayesian synthesis is designed primarily to provide *decision support* [17] where the review or synthesis is required to support a specific decision in a particular context. The three other methods (narrative, qualitative and quantitative) can be seen as largely providing *knowledge support* by integrating knowledge and thereby illuminating, but not directly informing, a range of potential decisions in a variety of contexts.

It is worth noting that many of the techniques suggested below were devised for either qualitative or quantitative synthesis and for analysing primary data. Like qualitative synthesis (on which some of the approaches draw), the methods for synthesising qualitative and quantitative research are in the early stages of development.

Narrative qualitative–quantitative synthesis

This approach is broadly as described under narrative synthesis above. Such work includes syntheses that attempt to integrate the findings of qualitative research with systematic reviews of quantitative literature, or meta-analyses of randomised trials. Harden *et al.*'s work combining a meta-analysis of trial data with a thematic analysis of qualitative studies to infer barriers and facilitators to healthy eating is a good example of this type of narrative-based synthesis of qualitative and quantitative research [18]. Narrative synthesis includes the example of meta-narrative mapping discussed in this chapter and would also encompass approaches such as Young's review of qualitative and quantitative literatures on illness behaviour [19]. This incorporated papers from 1973 onwards, covering a range of disciplinary approaches, including sociological, geographical and economic, to develop an integrated hierarchical model of illness behaviour.

Qualitative qualitative–quantitative synthesis

These approaches attempt to convert all available evidence into qualitative (i.e. textual) form, and then conduct the synthesis either using meta-ethnography or the qualitative cross-case type analytical methods described earlier in this chapter to produce new concepts or theories capable of explaining findings from different studies. A recent example of a qualitative approach, based on meta-ethnography, is an *interpretative synthesis* that examined a large literature on access to health care described by Dixon-Woods *et al.* [20].

Quantitative qualitative–quantitative synthesis

Quantitative approaches convert all evidence into quantitative (i.e. numerical) form. This can be done using techniques such as quantitative case survey – a process that uses a set of structured questions to extract 'observations' from either a set of case sites or separate studies that are then converted into numerical form and statistically analysed. For example, in the national evaluation of general practitioner 'total purchasing pilots' in the UK NHS, Mays *et al.* summarised a variety of mainly qualitative data from interviews and other sources to derive a quantitative 'score' for each total purchasing pilot site. This in turn reflected its ability to bring about service change elsewhere in the local NHS through its activities as a purchaser of health care [21]. It was then possible to relate the score to a range of characteristics of each pilot site in a quantitative analysis to begin to explain the relative success of the different pilots.

Another quantitative approach to synthesising qualitative and quantitative evidence is to use content analysis – a technique for categorising the data into themes that can then be counted and converted into frequencies to identify dominant issues across a number of studies.

Bayesian synthesis

This approach applies the principles of Bayesian analysis to synthesis. The data from multiple studies are converted into quantitative form and pooled for analysis and modelling. Bayesian synthesis is designed mainly for *decision support* where a review aims to support a specific decision. This approach can be useful because it has the capacity to incorporate sources such as expert or public opinion as well as qualitative research evidence into modelling/analysis. One example of a synthesis that used this approach is a study using qualitative and quantitative evidence to assess factors affecting uptake of immunisation [22]. This used the findings from qualitative studies of immunization uptake to inform a prior distribution (a numerical ranking of factors affecting immunisation uptake from individual studies). These prior probabilities were combined with probabilistic data extracted from quantitative studies and analysed together to identify and gauge the importance of a wider range of factors linked to uptake than either the qualitative or quantitative literatures could have provided alone.

Concluding remarks

The science of synthesis is evolving and many of the methods described in this chapter have only recently been applied to health and health care research evidence. Ultimately the choice of synthesis approach should relate to both the specific aim of the review and the nature of the available evidence. If only qualitative evidence is available or required, then one of the methods for qualitative synthesis described above may be appropriate. If a combination of qualitative and quantitative evidence is desired, it may be worth exploring the other approaches outlined, with the caveat that these are perhaps even less well developed than narrative synthesis, meta-ethnography or cross-case analysis. For qualitative–quantitative synthesis it may be that more than one approach will be required (as demonstrated in a number of reviews of qualitative and quantitative research undertaken by the Evidence for Policy and Practice Information and Co-ordinating Centre (EPPI-Centre) at the University of London, Institute of Education [23,24]).

In general, as with the methods used in primary research, the methods for synthesis should be explicit and transparent, but the key stages should be seen as flexible, pragmatic and iterative rather than strictly sequential. Inevitably, syntheses of complex bodies of evidence, whether solely qualitative, or combining qualitative and quantitative evidence, require experience and judgement on the part of the researchers.

Further reading

Dixon-Woods M, Agarwal S, Jones D, Young B & Sutton A. Synthesising qualitative and quantitative evidence: a review of possible methods. *Journal of Health Services Research and Policy* 2005; **10**: 45–53.

Mays N, Pope C & Popay J. Systematically reviewing qualitative and quantitative evidence to inform management and policy making in the health field. *Journal of Health Services Research and Policy* 2005; **10**(Suppl 1): 6–20.

References

1. Chalmers I & Altman DG. *Systematic Reviews*. BMJ Books, London, 1995.

2. Harden A, Garcia J, Oliver S *et al.* Applying systematic review methods to studies of people's views: an example from public health research. *Journal of Epidemiology and Community Health* 2004; **58**: 794–800.

3. Garcia J, Bricker L, Henderson J *et al.* Women's views of pregnancy ultrasound: a systematic review. *Birth* 2002; **29**: 225–250.

4. Hammersley M. *What's Wrong with Ethnography?* Routledge, London, 1992.

5. Pound P, Britten N, Morgan M *et al.* Resisting medicines: a synthesis of qualitative studies of medicine taking. *Social Science and Medicine* 2005; **61**: 133–155.

6. Evans D. Database searches for qualitative research. *Journal of the Medical Library Association* 2002; **3**: 290–293.

7. Shaw RL, Booth A, Sutton AJ *et al.* Finding qualitative research: an evaluation of search strategies. *BMC Medical Research Methodology* 2004; **4**: 5.

8. Dixon Woods M, Fitzpatrick R & Roberts K. Including qualitative research in systematic reviews: problems and opportunities. *Journal of Evaluation in Clinical Practice* 2001; **7**: 125–133.

9. Campbell R, Pound P, Pope C *et al.* Evaluating meta-ethnography: a synthesis of qualitative research on lay experiences of diabetes and diabetes care. *Social Science and Medicine* 2003; **56**: 671–684.

10. www.ccsr.ac.uk/methods/projects/posters/popay.shtml

11. Greenhalgh T. Meta-narrative mapping: a new approach to the synthesis of complex evidence. In: Hurwitz B, Greenhalgh T & Skultans V, eds. *Narrative Research in Health and Illness.* BMJ Publications, London, 2004.

12. Miles MB & Huberman AM. *Qualitative Data Analysis: An Expanded Sourcebook.* SAGE, London, 1994.

13. Yin R. *Case Study Research, Design and Methods.* Applied Social Research Methods Series, vol. 5. SAGE, Thousand Oaks, 1984.

14. Noblit G & Hare R. *Meta-Ethnography: Synthesising Qualitative Studies.* SAGE, Newbury Park, CA, 1988.

15. Britten N, Campbell R, Pope C, Donovan J, Morgan M & Pill R. Using meta ethnography to synthesise qualitative research: a worked example. *Journal of Health Services Research and Policy* 2002; **7**(4): 209–215.

16. Mays N, Pope C & Popay J. Systematically reviewing qualitative and quantitative evidence to inform management and policy making in the health field. *Journal of Health Services Research and Policy* 2005; **10**(Suppl 1): 6–20.

17. Dowie J. The Bayesian approach to decision making. In: Killoran A, Swann C & Kelly M, eds. *Public Health Evidence: Changing the Health of the Public.* Oxford University Press, Oxford, 2006 (forthcoming).

18. Harden A, Garcia J, Oliver S *et al.* Applying systematic review methods to studies of people's views: an example from public health research. *Journal of Epidemiology and Community Health* 2004; **58**: 794–800.

19. Young JT. Illness behaviour: a selective review and synthesis. *Sociology of Health and Illness* 2004; **26**: 1–31.
20. Dixon Woods M, Kirk D, Agarwal S *et al.* Vulnerable groups and access to health care: a critical interpretative synthesis. A report for the National Co-ordinating Centre for NHS Service Delivery and Organisation R&D (NCCSDO) www.sdo.lshtm.ac.uk/pdf/access_ dixon-woods_finalcopyedited.pdf
21. Goodwin N, Mays N, McLeod H, Malbon G, Raftery J, on behalf of the Total Purchasing National Evaluation team (TP-NET). Evaluation of total purchasing pilots in England and Scotland and implications for primary care groups in England: personal interviews and analysis of routine data. *British Medical Journal* 1998; **317**: 256–259.
22. Roberts KA, Dixon-Woods M, Fitzpatrick R, Abrams KR & Jones DR. Factors affecting the uptake of childhood immunisation: a Bayesian synthesis of qualitative and quantitative evidence. *Lancet* 2002: **360**: 1596–1599.
23. Oliver S. Making research more useful: integrating different perspectives and different methods. In: Oliver S & Peersman G, eds. *Using Research for Effective Health Promotion*. Buckingham Open University Press, 2001: 167–179.
24. Lumley J, Oliver S & Waters E. *Smoking Cessation Programs Implemented During Pregnancy*. The Cochrane Library Issue 3. Oxford: Update Software, 1998.

Index

access, to setting, 6, 17, 19, 22,
    35–6, 54, 56, 75, 83, 88,
    95–7, 104, 108, 149
action research, 121–9
    contribution, 124–5
    democracy in, 123–4
    description, 121–2
    in health care, 126–9
    participation, 122
    types, 125
analysis, *see also individual entries*,
    96–8, 137–8
    and writing up, 28
    and data, 65, 73, 88–9
analytic induction, 77
anonymity, 53–5
antirealism, 84–6
axial coding, 71

Bayesian synthesis, 148, 149–50
business process re-engineering,
    117

CA, *see* conversation analysis
CAQDAS (computer assisted
    qualitative data analysis
    software) packages, 74–5
case studies, 112–19
    case study research, 112–14
    comparisons, 116
    design, 114–18
    multiple methods, advantage,
        116
    site selection, 115
    theoretical sampling, 115
categories, 69
charting, 73
coding, 37, 66, 70–1, 76, 89

'collaborative spirals', in action
    research, 123
comparison, 71, 87, 95, 113,
    116–17, 127, 146–7
complementarity, 107
computer assisted analysis, 75
confidentiality
    ethical issue, 55–8
    problems in, 57
consensus development
    methods, 132–40
    analysis, 137–8
    approach, 138–40
    Delphi surveys, 134–5
    group meetings, 136–7
    nominal group techniques,
        134
    participant selection, 135–6
    practical issues, 135–7
    reasons for using, 132–3
    types, 133–4
constant comparison, 71
content analysis, 66, 149
conversation analysis, 43–51
    antibiotic prescribing decisions
        in, 48–9
    applications, 46–50
    in health care setting, 44–6, *see
        also separate entry*
    conduct, 44–6
    of audio-taped material, 64
    of everyday conversation, 50
    patient's/carer's perspective,
        47
    relevance, 43–4
    principles, 44
covert research, 36
crystallization, in mixed
    methods, 107